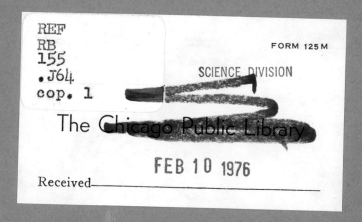

The Invisible Chain

The *INVISIBLE*

Elizabeth
Jolly, M.D.

CHAIN:

Diseases passed on by Inheritance

NELSON-HALL nh CHICAGO

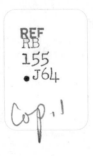
To Kay

ISBN: 0–911012–26–5

Library of Congress Card Number: 72-80166

Nelson-Hall Company, Publishers
325 W. Jackson Blvd., Chicago, Ill. 60606

Manufactured in the United States of America

Contents

I. To Kill a Myth   1

II. Diabetes   15

III. Arthritis   31

IV. Disorders of Vision   53

V. The Anemias   73

VI. Mental Illness   95

VII. Rheumatic Fever   111

VIII. Epilepsy   121

IX. The Rh Factor   139

X. Birth Defects   151

XI. Mental Retardation   165

XII. Of Universal and Elusive Maladies   179

XIII. Tomorrow through the Keyhole   193

Index   215

I

To Kill a Myth

SOMEWHERE BACK IN the pre-dawn hours of the human birthday nature slipped, committing a chemical error of the minutest proportions—and for the pre-human infant in whom the change occurred, as well as for his descendents, things were never again to be the same. Whatever the nature of the change, it ultimately ousted him from that primitive fraternity to which he had belonged and set him on a lonely journey up the long, erratic path that was to lead— slip-up by slip-up on nature's part—to modern man.

Since nature is hardly infallible of course, such occasional slip-ups are bound to occur. It is fortunate, in fact, that they do, for if nature never erred in repeating herself, life on earth would look today exactly as it did a billion or so years ago.

It is just such errors, as a matter of fact, that allow for evolution. Occurring in the blueprints, so to speak, by which life is shaped, in those miniscule units of heredity called "genes," they are responsible for the loss or the face-lifting of genes grown passé, for the equally accidental creation of new ones, for the increasingly complex creatures that these gene changes bring about—and for the evolving of man himself, with his bald body, his intelligence, his diabetes, his musical genius and his allergies.

Once such accidents occur, however, the die is cast. Once a gene is altered, all things thereafter built along its specifications will show the change. Let a builder overlook a detail on his blueprint and the structure he creates will be different, for either the better or the worse, from what the architect had prescribed. That is no fault of the blueprint, however, for it is still a valid prescription of what the architect envisioned. An error in the blueprint itself, on the other hand, would be a totally different story.

Let nature err in satisfying the blueprint instructions within a fertilized human egg—by providing it with, say, an infected womb—and the resulting damage to the infant will have no effect on his blueprint specifications, for the fault lay in the construction, not in the architectural design. And since it is only the "blueprint," the genes themselves, that is, that thread one generation to the next, it goes without saying that none of whatever damage this infant suffers as a result of nature's error will visit upon his descendents.

But let nature err in making a replica of that half of a parent's genes that are included in an egg or sperm, and the resulting infant, for better or for worse, has no escape from the dictates of that change. Dictates, incidentally, which any of his offspring who inherit the altered gene or genes must likewise follow.

Since the change occurs in the blueprint itself, this altered plan is at once established as the new order of a generations-long day.

By and large, nature carries out her work with an amazing degree of accuracy, and the marvel is she makes as *few* mistakes as she does. When she does slip-up, it is never intentional, never premeditated. And having erred, she carries on without ever a second thought, abiding by the dictates of the new order with at once the same indifference and the same diligence she had employed in carrying out the old.

Whether these little accidents will be good or bad for the host, therefore, is as purely random as tossing dice, with the estimated odds stacking up like this: ninety-nine bad effects to one good to an unknown number of neutrals. In other words, if the estimates are right, only one out of a hundred accidents—ignoring the neutral changes, those that neither help nor harm —is likely to put its host in a better position than he was before. The other ninety-nine changes penalize their hosts instead.

Now such changes, or *mutations* as they are called, happen only to individuals. But they can, eventually at least, "happen" also to a species. A really injurious change will not proliferate in a species, of course, because the individual in whom it occurs usually either dies or fails to procreate, and the problem ends there. If a mutation presents its host with a distinct *advantage* over the others of his group, however, he will likely live better and longer than the others. Thus he will

tend to have more offspring too, many of whom will
inherit from him the same advantage brought about
by the same mutant gene. Sooner or later, therefore,
his kind will begin to outnumber the others, and perhaps within only a few hundred thousand years or so,
his descendents will have either replaced the "old-
fashioned" type or left it behind and gone off somewhere to form a new tribe, or a new species.

These changes that result in new species, represent
the essence of evolution.

It is only when nature "mutates" the environment
instead of the individual that *extinction* occurs. For it
is only by the grace of the environment that a gene, or
the trait it determines, maintains its beneficial status.

If the species above, the new one, should ever
suffer an unfavorable environmental change, it is going
to be in trouble. Its special new trait, for example,
might have been a bill for catching fish that has en-
abled its members not only to live better but, over the
millennia, to come to depend on fish. A dependence
which could leave it in dire straits if, some time
later, due to sudden drought, all the fish-bearing rivers
and lakes began to dry up. Unless the drought were to
end before the species dwindled to an unsustainable
level, or unless nature just happened to make another
slip-up in just the right place, the handwriting on the
wall would spell extinction.

On the other hand, so long as the environment
continues to allow the trait to work to the species'
advantage, it will be all right. And that, as far as we
know, has been the lucky lot to date of most of the
plants and animals alive today.

In spite of her lack of bias in mutational affairs, nature is not 100 percent random in the errors that she makes, for certain mutations have a way of cropping up more often than others. Some genes seem to be simply more "slippery" than others to handle, or a little more fragile, or have a slightly greater affinity for the wrong kind of chemicals. At any rate, nature certainly does commit the same error twice, and thrice, and in the case of *some* mutations so often that one begins to suspect certain genes of being scandalously unstable.

For example, the most common form of *muscular dystrophy,* a disease largely limited to boys, is caused by a change of some sort in one of the genes assigned the job of seeing to it that muscles function normally. Perhaps this gene is a relative newcomer on the evolutionary scene and nature has therefore had less experience in its handling. In any event, in attempting to pass it on, intact, from one generation to the next, her accident rate is shocking. For she allows it to mutate so often, it is claimed, that a third of all boys who suffer from muscular dystrophy do so as a result of fresh mutations in themselves, not because they have inherited a mutant gene already present in the family.

Even genes that have been kicking around in evolutionary history for a long time are not necessarily immune to natural accidents. One can only speculate in what primeval forest and in what kind of ancient animal, a semi-catastrophe of another sort first occurred. This unknown soldier of an unknown species in the battle of evolution bore the marks of an error nature was to make time and again in mammals of all descriptions, including man: gross dwarfing of the extremities.

True, this kind of defect is not a painful one. Nor does it seem, directly, to affect the health of its host. *Indirectly,* however, it has all the potential of being catastrophic, for it is not a trait that augurs well for the survival either of the individual or—via his off-spring—of the altered gene. In the primeval days of our unknown soldier's existence, the deformed extremities must have been a critical handicap in his runnings-about for food. Or, conversely, in his runnings-about to keep from becoming food for some other kind of creature.

If his defect were not severe enough to keep him out of the competition altogether, it very likely put him at a telling disadvantage in his territorial struggles with the other members of his species. And without a mating ground, his chance of coming by a mate and, subsequently, progeny would have been reduced if not outright destroyed.

With so glum an outlook, how did the dwarfing gene keep itself going in sufficient numbers, in sufficient species, to become commonly recognized and properly categorized—as it is today by physicians and veterinarians alike—as *achondroplastic dwarfism?* Nature simply makes this same genetic mistake just often enough in new individuals to make up for the dwarfing genes that die, so to speak, with their hosts.

Of course, there are many kinds of mutations which nature rarely makes. And there are certain mutations that she is so unlikely to commit that they have occurred perhaps only a handful of times in evolutionary history.

Huntington's chorea, whose victims are given to spasmodic motions and incoordination, is an uncommon disease of man caused by a faulty gene whose original mutation nature so rarely repeats that most of the 10,000 cases in America today probably stem from only a dozen different ancestors. Not that nature could not make the same mistake anew, but since she so rarely does, the chances are overwhelming that anyone who develops this disease does so because he has inherited the abnormal gene from one or the other of his parents.

Nor does nature appear to be necessarily committed to her own directives. There seem to be instances of erasures, so to speak, of nature backtracking on herself. At least a few of her creations, at any rate, seem to be on shaky grounds. Unlike the highly stable if fearsome H. chorea gene, for example, that pursues an unrelenting course through the generational waves, some genes seem possessed of a little stagefright when cast in a mutant role. For they have a way of simply disappearing some acts later, possibly by slipping into different roles again, into further mutations as it were, or possibly by reverting back to their original, normal states.

In humans, for instance, there occurs a defect due to a mutant gene which the critic, long before the curtain falls, must conclude has been miscast. It is dominant enough in performing its role, asserting itself in every generation, and demonstrates versatility aplenty—unless that versatility, perhaps, is really only the reflection of some inconsistency, some weakness in its behavior, a clue to its ultimate failure after all. For in one individual it will show itself as only a few cream-and-coffee-colored, dime-sized freckles, while in someone else—a daughter maybe or a brother—it will literally cover the body with tumors and spots. And in another person still, perhaps the child of the family, it may put in a hushed appearance only, having nothing at all to say beyond the emptiness in the child's eyes, the wandering inexpressions of a silenced mind.

The defect produced by this unpredictable gene has been called, for want of a simpler name, *neurofibromatosis*. The condition is not at all uncommon but fortunately neither is it commonly severe. Perhaps then the mutant gene does not really have her heart in the play.

Regardless, though, the critic was right. The gene does seem to be miscast, for often, six or seven acts later, six or seven generations after her impromptu entrance, the defect disappears. And the play goes on, precisely as it had before she assumed her mutant role. So, where did she go? Her very absence should cause the genetic applecart to veer at least a little, should be noticeable in some way in the play itself. Unless—just possibly—she has not disappeared at all, and the critic, straining in the still dim stagelights of our young genetic knowledge, strives to see her faint resemblance on some older, more familiar face, some better-behaved, more permanent member of the cast, re-entering suddenly—as in a one-shot Jekyll and Hyde affair —after some brief absence from the stage.

So there are unstable actors and there are stable ones.

There are mutations whose effects are disastrous—for an individual or for a species—as well as mutations which are so minor in their effect as not to make one noticeable bit of difference to their hosts.

There are common mutations and there are rare ones. And then there are the *very* rare mutations. In fact, we must probably assume there are some which are so very unlikely they have yet to occur. And this may be grounds more for hope than despair.

When all is said and done, it is nature's capacity to err that provides a species—and the human species is no exception—with the variation it needs to survive. The more variation within a species, that is, the greater the number of forms and sizes and shapes of its individuals, the better its chance of survival. Any change in the environment that threatens one variety will not necessarily threaten all. The more shapes and forms that a species comes in, as a matter of fact, the more likely it is that at least one variation will allow those who possess it to survive in a new situation. The existence of varieties assures, therefore, the perpetuation of the species. In the case of our fish-eating friend with the improved bill, for example, species extinction might never have threatened had a few of his brethren maintained the ability to exist without fish.

A mutation, then, or the trait it results in, is good, bad or indifferent in only a *relative* sense. It may be good for its host today and quite something else a few generations later. Obviously, of course, the opposite may also occur.

Now concerning "bad" and "good" heredity, there are three or four myths kicking about—mega-myths if one is to judge by the number of people who believe in them—that need to be exploded.

One myth is the belief that a disease is a disease is a disease. Actually, there is no such thing as a disease at all, except in a relative sense. If an individual has trait X and trait X affects his health adversely, then for him, in that given environment, indeed the trait *is* a disease. But the trait cannot be called a disease in itself, for there is no saying in what new environment, in which one of his descendents, it may become a virtue, possibly even the key to his survival.

This concept is abstract, of course. Moreover, one might point to the ability to develop kidney stones or varicose veins, for example, as at no time in history having served any useful purpose. The concept is still valid, however. For the past is hardly synonymous with forever, and no trait has yet been tried, let alone found guilty, in all possible environments.

Take the dachshund, for example. Specifically, take the original dachshund from whom the breed was developed. He may have looked like a frankfurter to his long-legged litter mates and mother, but to his opportunistic owner the dog's peculiar proportions seemed made to order for hunting badgers in their burrows. The owner thereupon set about the business of arranging such in-breedings as were needed to establish a pure line of these unusual little dogs. Though the dachshund is not often used for hunting badgers anymore, the trait does continue to work to his advantage, for it has come to endear him to dachshund lovers the world over.

Obviously then, the trait has been a feather in the cap of his well-being. And none of his champions, even the little dog himself, could care less that, like that unknown soldier in the primeval past, he is an achondroplastic dwarf.

Another common mega-myth concerns "inherited disease." There is simply no such thing. The words imply in the first place that there are diseases which can be caused by heredity alone and that is absolutely not true. Indirectly, they also imply that there are some diseases in which heredity plays no role at all and that, of course, is likewise false. No one exists in a vacuum, and neither do one's genes. Like individuals, genes must have some environment with which to interact or they are nothing at all. By the same token, what the environment does to a creature depends on the latitudes allowed by that creature's genes.

Every schoolchild knows that measles is caused by a virus. So what can possibly be hereditary about something so obviously environmental? Simply this: in order to get measles one must be susceptible to the virus. And susceptibility, after all, is determined by the genes. Rabbits, for example, are immune to the disease. And the only real difference between rabbits and men is genetic, of course. The fact that all human beings are susceptible to measles does not make it one whit *less* genetic. It simply means that *all* human beings possess the genes that make for vulnerability.

At the other extreme are diseases like Huntington's chorea. Sooner or later everyone possessing the H. chorea gene develops the disease, but no one who lacks the gene ever does so. What can possibly be environmental, then, about something so obviously inherited?

The self-same argument of interaction between environment and genes holds in reverse. Without an environment with which to interact, no gene can have expression. Programmed only to say a certain word, its voice depends entirely on those letters of the alphabet the environment happens to supply. The fact that 100 percent of persons with the H. chorea gene will develop the disease merely means that the environmental ingredients, whatever they are, are too universal to escape or too indispensable to life in general for anyone to do without. Perhaps the activating agent is every bit as ubiquitous as such other veterans of our environment as oxygen, or water, or everyday stress and strain. Therefore, the case for an environmental co-villain is not lessened by one iota.

All the same, "hereditary disease," as an expression, is a handy term for a disorder which develops only in those who host a given miscreant gene or genes. And as long as one keeps in mind the above limitations of environment and genes, this usage of the term seems fair.

Still another myth guards the closet wherein the family skeleton is kept. It has to do with the illusion that an inherited disease is a reflection—if not an out and out stain—on the family tapestry. Such an illusion, however, is readily dispelled by the knowledge that untoward mutations are purely happenstance affairs, as is the eenie-meenie-minie method by which they filter down the generations. Accidents that result in disease are no more deserved than those mutations that result in musical genius, say, or fine strong teeth, or a long life span.

On an average, it is estimated, each of us hosts about a dozen undesirable genes, such as those whose expression results in mental retardation, blindness, deafness or the like. He without a patently inherited disease, then, does not necessarily harbor any *fewer* undesirable genes than persons *with* heredity problems. It is simply that those bad actor genes he does possess are not particularly assertive, tend not to express themselves unless backed up by a partner gene with the same adverse intent. Fortunately for the species, a good many of our undesirable genes do tend to be of this retiring nature. Thus, a person can merrily carry any number of such genes, pretty much in blissful unawareness, as long as each of those undesirable genes has a better-intentioned partner. Which is to say, as long as a person does not inherit from *both* of his parents the *same* defective gene he shows no signs of any adverse genes of the retiring sort he carries. And it is not too likely that he will inherit two defective genes of the same pair, because the storehouse of relatively faulty genes from which each of us gets to select the dozen we have coming is so vast.

Finally, there is the myth—whose multitudinous subscribers include a few people who really ought to know better—that little can be done about a faulty gene. True, no one yet has the technical know-how to do any downright engineering on the genes themselves.

But there are many ways of thwarting the acts of a
culprit other than by attacking him directly. Just to
know he is there, for example, may help to give one
the upper hand in things, especially if one finds him
out before he has a chance to wreak much havoc. For
it is sometimes possible, depending on the kind of culprit he is, to change his would-be felonies to mis-
demeanors, or even, in the case of certain disorders, to
deprive him actually of the wherewithal for doing anything mischievous at all.

As a matter of fact, hardly a month goes by without someone's having added to the armory of scientific
weapons for holding such culprits in check.

And that, basically, is what this book is all about—
the devious and not-so-devious devices that man has
invented, in an evolution of his own making, to control
those ills spawned by various misprints in the blueprint specifications of the human design.

In short, this is a book about those common hereditary ills whose chances of appearing in other family
members can be fairly well predicted and whose preventions, partial or complete, are already off the draft-
ing board and in production, so to speak.

It is a book not so much for the afflicted as for
those who are about to be, today, tomorrow, or a decade
hence. It is for the parents, the brothers and the sisters,
the sons and the daughters of those with inherited ills—
for the whole of that vulnerable kinfolk population
which, sooner or later, by virtue of one kind of hereditary ill or another, most of us end up joining.

II

Diabetes

CONSIDERING THE ANTIQUITY of diabetes and the wide variety of animals that fall victim to it, horses and hamsters, cats and dogs, mice and men—considering, too, that its tendency to run in families is so obvious that even the ancients, who knew nothing about genes, knew it was inherited—one would think that we, who by now know so much about genes, would have a crystal clear picture of precisely *how* it is inherited.

But we do not.

We do not know, for example, whether the gene is the retiring sort that must be inherited from *both* of one's parents to produce the disease or if it is so domineering that only the contribution of a single parent is needed. We cannot even be sure that diabetes is not a *many*-gene effect.

If our assumption that diabetes is a single disease is erroneous, that in itself, of course, could account for our failure, to date, to ferret out the responsible gene or genes. It is certainly not inconceivable that more than one kind of underlying defect could lead to diabetes, each defect caused by a different gene, each inherited in its own way, each having nothing in common with any of the others except for the end result: that block of signs and symptoms we label "diabetes."

As a matter of fact there is some pith to the suspicion that not all diabetes *is* one disease. Some studies suggest, for example, that the relatives of persons who develop the disease in childhood have a greater chance of developing diabetes than the relatives of those who do not become diabetic until later in life. Such a finding, if correct, certainly could result if juvenile diabetes differed from the adult disease in the kind of gene or genes that produced it.

The age at which diabetes develops, however, is a wobbly basis at best for the separation of cases. In an adult the disease occasionally behaves in the erratic fashion common to the juvenile form, while in a youngster it sometimes exhibits the more stable behavior of the adult-type disease. Until separate genetic factors can be identified, then, and persons with diabetes separated accordingly, we must study the general group of all diabetics to get some notion of the heritability of this disease.

With all their limitations, however, such studies provide us with something much better than nothing at all, considering the blatant tendency of diabetes in general to recur in those families in which it has already put in an appearance.

And what do such studies reveal?

How close do they tell us the disease must approach one's own perch on the family tree before it portends for him a risk enough above the average to justify his taking some precautionary action?

What are one's future chances of getting, or escaping, the disease if it is his aunt who is diabetic? Or one of his parents? Or *both* his parents, perhaps?

How high—as the risks of developing diabetes go—is "high"?

Or what, to begin with, is the "average" risk if it is the average risk that, by comparison, makes "high" what it is?

Now these are fair enough questions, but if their answers are to be helpful, they need a perspective in which to be viewed. And that perspective includes the fact that the average individual's chance of developing diabetes at some time during the normal life span is astonishingly high. About one-fourth of all people, it is said, give a positive family history for diabetes. Are able, that is, to recall some blood relative who has or had the disease, and since many people know little, and maybe care less, about their relatives past the first cousin category, this means the cases they *are* aware of come pretty close to home in most such instances. Moreover, there is nothing niggardly about the frequency of the disease in the total population. No less than 3 percent of people in the United States—one out of every thirty-three is said to be affected. And that does not include those cases still in such an early stage that they have yet to develop symptoms.

For *any* disease that is quite a record.

True, there are populations around that are almost

totally nondiabetic. Among the Eskimos, for example, documented cases of diabetes can be counted on the fingers of one hand. There are groups where the opposite is true, like the Pima Indians of the American Southwest, among whom diabetes is so very common that by the age of thirty-five, over half the population has at least its earliest signs. But these are the extremes, and while the rate has been reported to be slightly lower in Orientals than in Europeans, for most of the populations on earth the 3 percent figure is probably pretty valid.

So very common is diabetes, as a matter of fact, that there is hardly anyone who fails to recognize it as a disease not to be taken lightly. And therein lies a most compelling sort of enigma. Things that are severe and things that are common make strange bedfellows, at least as far as hereditary diseases are concerned.

The more severe a disease is, of course, the more likely it is to incapacitate, if not destroy, its host. If this occurs before the individual reaches child-bearing age, there is little or no opportunity of his passing on the disease-causing gene or genes to the next generation. Such genes, then, tend to die with their hosts. Under conditions such as these, nature would have to produce new mutations at an unheard-of clip in order to keep the particular disease from being anything but a rarity.

Granted, today's young diabetics, under treatment, by and large survive right through the procreative years. But only since the discovery of insulin—not much more than half a century ago—has this been true. Diabetes, on the other hand, is a disease of such antiquity that it undoubtedly made its appearance in pre-man's genetic blueprint long before his evolutionary ouster from that primitive fraternity forced him down the path to contemporary man. And in that interval— from well over a million years ago right up to the present, the last sixty years being an almost insignificant drop in the bucket of living time—diabetic youngsters did not live to procreate. And the procreative adult who developed the disease did not live long enough thereafter to have another child.

As an evolutionary rule, the most prolific genes are those that confer the biggest favors on their hosts. By the reverse token, the least prolific genes are those that do the most disservice.

How then did diabetes, in what gives all the appearances of having been a most flagrant taunting of this rule, achieve the seemingly impossible? With what kind of wheelings and dealings did it manage to achieve that state of evolutionary distinction known as "the commonplace"?

Almost certainly, once upon a time, diabetes did its host a favor of sorts.

But what kind of favor? And in what manner bestowed?

No one really knows.

Perhaps, as has often been suggested, the answer lies in the tendency of diabetic girls to become fertile at a younger age than their nondiabetic peers. This, of course, would hardly have been of consequence to diabetic girls in eons past, for without treatment, survival was limited and pregnancy, if it occurred at all, was doomed. But this fertility advantage is not limited to girls who are frankly diabetic. It occurs in *pre-*

diabetic girls as well—girls who have all the genetic wherewithal for developing diabetes but have not done so yet. And while such girls have a greater tendency to problem pregnancies than nondiabetic girls, their earlier fertility may more than compensate for any lack of fertility later in life, it is thought.

Given more years in which to procreate then, the pre-diabetic girl might well end up with proportionately more children than the girl who was not diabetic. Each succeeding generation, therefore, would contain proportionately more diabetic members. But this, by itself, could hardly account for today's marked prevalence of the disease.

As with any really good mystery the answer remains elusive enough to excite a little healthy cogitation. And so, now and then, one hears whisperings from the basements of science where theories brew, from the burbling vats of speculation yeasted with the bits and pieces of any and all findings that seem even remotely relevant.

In such ways are rare theories concocted, not the least plausible of which is a rather recent suggestion that in periods of famine the person with pre-diabetes possibly may have had an edge over the nondiabetic in terms of downright survival.

That early man had famines aplenty—particularly before he took to the planting of crops some one hundred centuries ago—is widely accepted. Of all the things that stalked him in those unarmored days of his early existence, starvation almost undoubtedly was one of the hardest to parry. An ability to withstand starving then may well have been a weapon at least as crucial to his survival as the club he used to ward off predators of other kinds.

Obviously, the greater one's ability to withstand starvation, the greater his chance of surviving any famine. Those with unusually great abilities—as might result, say, from a special kind of body chemistry— would, of course, have a telling survival advantage over those who lacked such a biochemical talent. By the time the famine abated, individuals with the special ability could therefore be expected to make up a greater percent of the population than before, by virtue of the death of many of their less-advantaged comrades. And if this special ability, this special kind of body chemistry, were *inherited,* obviously there would be a proportionate increase, come the next generation, in the responsible genes.

But what evidence is there that pre-diabetes may have provided its hosts with such an ability?

Normally, when a man starves he more or less starves all over. The disadvantage of this, of course, is that it puts the different parts of him—for example, his muscles, his liver and his brain—into fierce competition for what little fuel is available from the storehouses of his own body. As a matter of fact, such organs become so busy competing for any and all sugar they can get hold of that both the liver and the muscles fail to notice another nearby fuel which, although not refined enough for the brain, would do them nicely.

Ironically, according to the hypothesis, the metabolic "defect" that causes diabetes may have arbitrated, to the starving man's advantage in famines past, this destructive competition among his organs. For, as it happens, this defect, this "special body chemistry" as it were, is a prolific producer of fatty acids from the body's own storehouse of fat. Fatty acids in sufficient amounts do several things. They handcuff the liver, so to speak, at least as far as using sugar is concerned, forcing the liver to direct its talents toward the *making* of sugar instead. In return they provide the liver with a little of the raw material for doing so.

Arbitrating this chemical war one step further, these excess fatty acids persuade the muscles to leave off sugar by offering themselves as an equally effective fuel, thereby assuring a maximum supply of sugar for the brain—and peace of a sort for all involved contestants.

True, under ordinary circumstances this sort of thing can well get a man into trouble, and no one would say that the man with pre-diabetes was any better off for being on the verge of starving to death. He simply may have been better off than his nondiabetic comrades at such times, for in the face of death by starvation his defect might have been exactly what the medicine man would have ordered.

Whether this hypothesis must eventually be dumped down the drain in the brew cellars of science or given some permanent place upstairs in the gallery of facts, its assumption remains valid: in some way, in some place, in some bygone time, diabetes was not all bad.

In no other way can one account more logically for a disease so prevalent that the average man or woman's chance of developing it is just about one out of thirty.

This figure is a bit of an artifact, of course, for the *average man* is less of a man than a fiction. He is an arithmetic result, the average of *all* men, *real* men, mixed together. It is entirely possible, then, depending on what characteristic one is measuring, to find that only a fraction of real men—maybe only a few, maybe no one at all—will fit exactly on that line that marks the average. Some, many, or all real men will be off to the sides. While averages are downright handy when one is looking at groups, then, they are not as useful in making predictions about an individual.

Thus, there are undoubtedly many individuals whose chances of developing diabetes are less than one out of thirty. There may be those homing in around that average mark, and there will be many, like the close blood kin of those with the disease, whose chances run the gamut from slightly above the average to something approaching a certainty.

Even for relatives, however, the chance of getting diabetes must be taken as applying to the average individual in any relationship group. For if diabetes is a mix of separate genetic disorders, its chance of developing in the offspring, say, of a diabetic parent may not necessarily be the same for the offspring of *every* diabetic parent.

Moreover, the figures as they are given below apply to one's chance of developing the disease during a life span of something like eighty years. Obviously that chance will be reduced from birth if one is slated, at age thirty say, to fall in the well, for not only has *he* been cheated out of another fifty years but so has his chance of developing the disease. Since, given his druthers, however, he would surely have preferred to be around to go on worrying about developing diabetes, the eighty-year risks are perhaps the more meaningful after all.

The risks for various relatives run something like this: with a diabetic parent or sibling (brother or sister, that is) one's chance of getting the disease is roughly one out of five. The same risk applies to the parent of a diabetic child.

The presence of the disease in a combination of such relatives does not imply a risk that is significantly greater, nor do additional cases in relatives more remote—so long as they are all on the *same* side of the family.

If the disease is not that exclusive, however, the story is somewhat different. For example, while affected grandparents, aunts, or uncles on one side only imply a risk that is only slightly greater than that prevailing in the general population, the occurrence of such affected relatives on *both* sides of the family makes one's risks one out of ten.

The risks increase to one out of three if that two-sided distribution by chance should include a diabetic parent.

There are even two situations in which one is less likely to escape than develop the disease. Should both of one's parents be diabetic, one's chance of developing the disease, given a full life span, is said to be nine out of ten, and greater than half before he is even forty.

The risk is likewise high among those who happen to have an affected identical twin. Where one twin is affected, so is the other, sooner or later, in nearly 100 percent of such pairs.

It goes without saying, of course, that these figures hold for blood relatives only. In-laws, step-relatives, and adoptions simply do not count.

Enough of figures except to repeat that those given here are artificially high. While not many of us will fall in the well at age thirty, some of the heft in these figures derives from what *would* have happened to certain individuals had they not succumbed to other things at seventy.

In short, these figures are not really scary. Rather, they are utopian in the sense that only under utopian conditions of health and longevity—the kind of conditions most of us would give our eye teeth to have— will, say, a full 20 percent of all the brothers and sisters of persons with diabetes actually develop the disease.

From a practical standpoint, of course, it is what one can *do* about such information that matters in the end. Knowing, for example, that one is a likely candidate for *any* disorder is not particularly helpful if such knowledge is productive only of insomnia. In the case of diabetes, worrying would be a pitiful waste of time, considering the means available for detecting and often preventing the disease before it becomes apparent.

There are, for example, rather reliable tests for identifying outwardly healthy people in whom the earliest silent changes of diabetes have just begun to occur, sometimes years before the onset of recognizable symptoms and the need for insulin treatment. Of these tests the most common is the *glucose tolerance test,* a technique designed to measure the amount of sugar in the blood over a period of time. Immediately after the ingestion of a large amount of sugar, both normal and diabetic persons show an increased blood sugar level. It is not so much a difference here that distinguishes them. The real distinction comes a couple of hours later when the blood sugar of the nondiabetic has already fallen to its original level while that of the diabetic—including the outwardly healthy person in whom the diabetic change is yet too early to result in symptoms—will still be sluggishly on its way down.

Now the test will not detect the individual in whom even those earliest changes have yet to occur, in the *pre*-diabetic, that is. For this reason it has been recommended that even if the test yields negative results, it should be repeated every five years in all close blood relatives of diabetic persons.

The onset of frank diabetes, it is often said, is not, after all, a signal of battle begun. It is rather the incontestable sign that the battle has already been waged, and lost. Such a defeat, if the truth were known, all too often could have been avoided.

It was no accident that the incidence of new cases throughout Europe was unusually low when, as a result of the war, the supplies of food were low, too. Neither was it any accident that when the war was over the replenishing of national larders was followed by so much diabetes all at once as to give the illusion of an almost-epidemic.

Today, simple weight control, the avoidance of obesity, is still the best all-around prevention of frank diabetic disease. Granted, it is a measure *everyone* would do well to follow, but for the *potential diabetic* it is crucial.

The *pre*-diabetic, of course, is included in this latter group. Or rather, since pre-diabetes is still, by definition, a state "too early to detect," one really ought to say the *presumed* pre-diabetic. Like the offspring, for example, of two diabetic parents. And those female relatives of a diabetic who give presumptive evidence of their likely pre-diabetic states by having ten-pound babies.

It would not be at all amiss, in fact, for safety's sake, to consider the avoidance of obesity crucial for *all* close relatives of diabetic persons—along, with any woman, whether related to a known diabetic or not, whose babies at birth weigh over ten pounds.

Once a glucose tolerance test yields positive results, of course, there is no question in the matter. For if the disease has developed to the point where the test can detect it, it is usually only a matter of time, in the absence of dietary caution, before the symptoms of frank diabetes appear.

On occasion, in addition to diet regulation, a physician may even prescribe one or another of those oral medications that are given at times to those in whom the frank disease is already fully established.

Our present knowledge of diabetes, of course, is far from complete. Though it is vastly greater than it was a half a century ago, it is vastly more sketchy, in all likelihood, than it will be a half a century hence, for by then, hopefully, we shall know what we do not know now. We shall have learned what the deep-down basic defect in diabetes really is, perhaps, down where the genes do their work, many action layers beneath the level of overt signs and symptoms, and the manner, perhaps, in which that defect is passed from one to the next generation.

We may, in fact, have discovered *several* kinds of basic defects, several different kinds of diabetes, as it were, each with a different degree and kind of heritability.

In all probability we shall know more about the nature—and therefore control—of those environmental agents that influence the behavior of diabetic genes.

There is every reason to believe that, sooner rather than later, we shall be able not only to detect pre-diabetes but to detect it in newborns, perhaps years before they are scheduled to develop frank diabetic disease. Take the recently reported finding, for example, that in pre-diabetic infants—so presumed because of two diabetic parents—the blood vessel walls seem to differ in structure from those of other infants. Results of other studies showing chemical differences between the insulins made by normal and diabetic individuals seem equally provocative.

Each finding in itself could be a new beginning, a crack in the door to some new room of unpredictable dimensions. Since only when we know a thing can we defend ourselves against it, each such finding increases the potential for better treatment and prevention.

As it is true of other diseases, so is it true of diabetes—more so, perhaps, considering the sophisticated chemistry in which its workings are enmeshed—that a clearer understanding of its abnormalities cannot help but give us, over the long haul, a clearer understanding of the whole human design. For diabetes, like all other human traits, is a part of that design. And though the disease is an exception in the sense that nondiabetes is the rule, it is from the exceptions to rules rather than from rules themselves that we learn—and in the learning become better able to cope with both.

III

Arthritis

IN THE PRIMEVAL mist of a bygone day an aging dinosaur stops at the foot of the slightest hillock, tries twice to shift his weight upward and, failing this, limps stiffly around it instead. In the musty light of a limestone shelter in Chapelle aux Saints, millennia-removed from today, a Neanderthal woman cushions a bear hide behind the shoulders of her man to ease the pain and, because he cannot chew, feeds him from her lips. In the bolder sunlight of some contemporary scene a German shepherd dog, bounding toward the sound of his master's voice, yelps suddenly and, stopping, commences to whimper.

Such is the antiquity of arthritis, such is the diversity of its victims.

Such is its enormous reach that the fingerprints of its one hand linger still on the fossil bones of dinosaurs while its other hand, even now, is pointing squarely at the bones of creatures as yet to be born.

Such is the versatility of this affliction that to be a victim—whether one swims, flies, or walks—requires merely the possession of joints.

Looking at the contemporary scene alone, considering the vulnerability imposed on man by his very jointedness, one is tempted to conclude that the most remarkable thing about arthritis after all is not that 15 percent of the human species suffer from some chronic form of it but that 85 percent of us manage not to.

One can begin to understand a little better, then, how the brewing potpourri of facts, theories, and beliefs concerned with arthritis has, in the short span of the human existence, become so highly spiced with misconceptions. Misconceptions, in particular, about the workings of heredity in the myriad disorders that one way or another expend their venom on the human joint.

Man, it must be admitted, has a compulsive bent for generalizing. A tendency so uncontrollable, at times, that he will conjure up an entire universe on the basis of a single sample, knowing full well, but blinded by his own enthusiasm to the fact, that the single sample may be a not very typical specimen. May be, by chance, as unrepresentative of its kind as was that prehistoric man unearthed in 1908 from his limestone grave in Chapelle aux Saints. And one wonders, in the queasiness of a post-enthusiasm hang-over, to what extent we have unjustly committed the image of the entire Neanderthal species to a stooping, bent-kneed stance, ignoring a little too zealously the possibility that the stooped frame was testimony neither to the sculpture of a whole species nor even to the intrinsic sculpture of that single prehistoric individual himself but simply to the fact that—like millions of others who currently share the same fate—he hurt.

With the same queasiness we survey the spicy potpourri of notions about arthritis itself and wonder, knowing the answer full well, how all the misconceptions came about.

The truth is relatively simple. Man over-generalizes and misconceptions are born.

Let us illustrate with lightning.

By anyone's odds, the chance of being struck by lightning is remote. The chance that any one family would have two such unfortunate accidents is even more remote. Take a large enough population, however, with a sprinkling of families in which lightning has already struck once, and sooner or later there will be a family counting its second victim.

No such family would be inclined to believe that being struck by lightning is hereditary, of course. But suppose now, rather than lightning, it had been rheumatoid arthritis that had struck. That self-same family might have difficulty controlling a conviction that something gene-deep was at work among them, even though rheumatoid arthritis is nowhere nearly so rare a predator as lightning. Even though rheumatoid arthritis is so very common that that same large population could yield many more twice- and thrice-hit families than lightning ever struck, all its victims are single-handedly selected by that one entity that has no axes to grind with any man—Chance.

It is such twice- and thrice-struck families, though, that one is most inclined to notice, and, noticing, to generalize upon without considering how much more numerous those families are with only one affected member.

Even rheumatologists now and then have fallen into this trap, awakened in the midnight of their scientific contemplations with that gnawing foreboding in their scientific bones that rheumatoid arthritis is a family affair.

But midnights, even long midnights, are a highly perishable phenomenon. And sooner or later, of course, dawn does come, concealing within it, true, the small dark embryo of yet another midnight, of another rash of questions yet to be answered, which the dawn itself begets.

And so rheumatoid arthritis is enjoying itself a dawn, after a long and troublesome night. And for whatever new questions the dawn may be provoking, it *has* brought light—that emanating from an increasing number of error-proofed studies which must convince even the skeptical that, in all likelihood, rheumatoid arthritis is a predominantly happenstance affair.

Such studies have not ruled out the possibility that in the very rare family heredity does play a significant role. But the evidence *for* this occurrence is primarily the lack of evidence *against* it. In any case, if they exist at all, such families would appear to be so few and so far between that even he with several arthritic relatives could fret more logically over his chance of slipping in the bathtub or forgetting on some crucial day to fasten the seat belt in his car.

Admittedly, earlier studies on rheumatoid arthritis did suggest inheritance. But these studies, through an inadvertent error in selection, were unduly weighted with families having two or more cases. The final result, then, was more or less destined to make rheumatoid arthritis look at least a *little* bit inherited. Under the same circumstances, it might be added, studies could be made to show that being struck by lightning was inherited, too.

But rheumatoid arthritis is only one of many different arthritic diseases, each distinct from the others in its cause, all of them wreaking some kind of havoc on the human joint. In this vast miscellany there *do* occur three kinds of arthritis which are relatively common and which show a predilection for the close blood kin of affected individuals: osteoarthritis, ankylosing spondylitis, and that long time favorite of medical chroniclers—the gout.

OSTEOARTHRITIS

It can be argued, of course, that osteoarthritis is a miscellany in itself, which is more of a fact than an argument, really, for the term encompasses that whole fraternity of disorders that bring about what are called "degenerative" changes in the joint.

The battlefields of osteoarthritis are vast. They are peopled with the aged, with the not-so-old whose joints reflect a little too precociously the wear-and-tear of life, with men and porpoises and birds, and German shepherds of most aristocratic stance, come to pay the piper for that extravagance—a veritable army on a

historic field strewn with the fossil reminders of dinosaur aches and pains. All of them victims of disorders
in which trauma probably plays a more important role
than heredity. In fact, trauma alone can produce osteoarthritis, as it not infrequently does, for example, in
laborers and athletes, or in anyone else whose joints
are subject to more than the usual amount of abuse.

The effects of heredity, on the other hand, are still
a subject of debate: Is the inherited vulnerability,
where it exists, a metabolic one, leading to chemical
abnormality of the joint tissue, or is it a purely mechan-
ical thing instead, with some individual joints simply
not having the right configuration to handle the load?

In view of the different disorders of hip and
spine and other diverse joints that make up osteoarthritis, it seems likely that both kinds of hereditary
effects occur. But in any case there is almost surely
still conspiracy with trauma.

Whatever contributions the genes make, however,
and granted they do make contributions, a sizable
predilection for the next-of-kin has been clearly
demonstrated in only one of the common kinds of
osteoarthritis: *Heberden's nodes.*

However unfamiliar its name, this disorder is
perhaps the most easily recognized of all forms of
osteoarthritis. This is the affliction that leaves so many
middle-aged and older women with those familiar
node-like swellings of the joints closest to the finger
tips.

Occasionally, Heberden's nodes are the direct
result of injury, but this occurs more often in men as
in an occasional baseball player or bowler. In such

cases the swelling tends to affect a single joint in contrast to the kind of Heberden's nodes with which we
are concerned here: arthritis not preceded by any clear-
cut history of injury, affecting more than one finger as
a rule, and as a rule affecting fingers only.

This rather specialized form of osteoarthritis gives
all the appearances of being caused by a single gene
which, while shy of expression in men, rarely *fails* to
assert itself in women.

For this reason, mothers, sisters, and daughters of
affected women could each be presumed to have a fifty-
fifty chance of developing Heberden's nodes, at least
by the age of seventy. By actual count, however, the
disorder appears to be no more than three times as common in such relatives as in women in the general population. This ratio could suggest any one of three different things: that the gene is not so assertive as we
thought; that many of the relatives observed were still
too young to be affected; or simply that there are a lot
of unrecognized genes for Heberden's nodes in the
general population. Regardless, there seems to be little
doubt that the close blood kin of affected women are
a particularly vulnerable group.

Since the culprit gene, even in this disorder, must
work hand-in-hand with some degree of trauma, such
high-risk women might be advised, as a perfectly bona
fide means of postponing the disorder and retarding its
course, to avoid abusing their hands. Since no one
abuses his hands deliberately, however, and since most
of us—by our occupations, by our dedications, or by
both—are committed in varying degrees to the use of
our hands, this kind of advice seems a little absurd.

Better perhaps for the woman at risk to bide her time, for she has at least an equal chance of never being affected at all. If and when she does develop symptoms, she still has time to modify the course of her affliction by minimizing unnecessary use of her hands. Moreover, she can derive a modicum of satisfaction from the fact that the disorder occasionally runs its entire course with no appreciable discomfort. And if she does experience discomfort from the disease, she can console herself with the knowledge that, though the swelling is permanent, the pain at least is not. The disease does burn itself out.

But the best of all reassurances, of course, will come simply from knowing that this affliction is rarely, if ever, a crippling disease.

So the most flagrantly inherited of all osteoarthritic disorders, as things turn out, is also one of the mildest.

As for other kinds of osteoarthritis—whatever their subtle obligation to heredity—it would finally appear that one's chance of affliction is determined not so much by the state of his kinship as by the state of his joints. The most susceptible among us seem to be those whose joints have already suffered a problem, such as a frank injury or a dislocation due, say, to faulty joint development, whether that faulty development is itself inherited or not.

Trauma of this kind, of course, is unlikely to have escaped the notice of its host. Like a red flag waving, it signals him to the need to practice a little discretion, like "living within" the limits of his joint, sparing the joint the added burdens of obesity and postural imperfections, keeping it limber without, in the process, adding further trauma.

For certain of osteoarthritis' potential victims at least, such common sense measures, if consistently taken, are probably enough to prevent the disease altogether. And if, in spite of the widespread application of such precautions, the incidence of arthritis continues to be high, it will not be because the measures are useless but because there are so very *many* of us in the vulnerable group.

After all, if one-fourth of all women and more than one-seventh of all men by the age of sixty-five have enough osteoarthritis to notice it, one can only conclude that trauma, like heredity, is a universal phenomenon, and that evolution has yet to endow us with the best of all possible joints.

Ankylosing Spondylitis

Unlike osteoarthritis, ankylosing spondylitis is a single disorder. And unlike rheumatoid arthritis, with which it is sometimes confused, it is very much an hereditary affair.

Not to be confused with osteoarthritis of the spine, ankylosing spondylitis is the disorder that characteristically leads to complete spinal rigidity, or "poker back," as it is called. The picture is rife with individual variation, of course. In some of its victims, the disease is at best half-hearted, never seeming to gain much momentum, occasionally giving up the ghost altogether before serious loss of spinal motion has occurred. In other cases, the disease descends with a fury, producing extreme deformity and poker-back in a few short years. The majority of its sufferers, however, fall anywhere in between.

Six people in every thousand, it is estimated, are susceptible to this disease. At that rate even the average village should contain a full-blown case or two.

Not nearly so common as osteoarthritis, ankylosing spondylitis has a way nonetheless of provoking recognition even in the smallest of children. To see a man bent over far enough nearly to touch his toes only to discover that he is there not to tie his shoes or to look for fallen pennies but simply because he no longer has any choice in the matter—to see a grown man imprisoned so by forces too invisible for a child's mind to understand is to grow up and grow old and still never forget it.

Invisible though they be, however, such forces are as real as the gene that masterminds them, and nearly as invincible. For this gene is aggressive enough to solo the show, to assert itself at the sacrifice of any expression to the contrary that might have been intended by the genetic partner-contribution of its owner's other parent.

Whether it is now and then forgetful, or persuaded into silence by some environmental agent, the gene for ankylosing spondylitis is not invariably given to expression. With what seems to smack of downright partiality, it is nine times more likely to keep silent if its host is a woman. As a matter of fact, only 10 percent of women who harbor the gene ever develop the disease. By contrast, 70 percent of its male hosts will sooner or later feel its effects.

What can be said, then, in the way of risks to relatives imposed by the now-aggressive, now-retiring behavior of this gene?

Since anyone who possesses the ankylosing spondylitis gene has a fifty-fifty chance of passing it on to each and every offspring, and since any child who *does* inherit it has either a 70 percent chance (if he is a son) or a 10 percent chance (if she is a daughter) of becoming affected, the risks are easily deduced.

Each son of an affected parent has one chance out of three of developing the disease. The same risk applies to the brother of a victim. Having both a parent and a sibling who are affected does not increase that risk.

The chance drops to one out of six for a boy whose closest affected relative is a grandparent or uncle on his mother's side. And his risk drops to one out of twenty if such affected relatives occur on his father's side instead—not because his father's family lacks any hereditary punch but simply because his father is far less likely to have inherited the gene without showing it. And if he does not have the gene, of course, he could not possibly have given it to his son.

By contrast, the chance that the daughter or sister of a patient will develop ankylosing spondylitis is about one out of twenty. Beyond that, a girl's chances pretty much pale into insignificance.

The parent, more likely a mother than a father, who carries the gene without showing it, is no less likely to have an affected offspring, of course, than the parent with full-blown disease. Moreover, if she has no affected relatives to tip her off, the appearance of ankylosing spondylitis in her son may come as a complete surprise. Such instances certainly do occur and there is no way of predicting them beforehand. But for any individual whose family contains no persons afflicted with ankylosing spondylitis, regardless of what other kinds of arthritis may plague them, the chance of this event is so slim—less than one in a thousand—as to make most other kinds of hazards a more logical concern.

When *both* parents harbor the gene for ankylosing spondylitis, sons may be at a risk as high as six out of ten, while the risk for daughters may run higher than one out of seven.

The real, most vulnerable targets for ankylosing spondylitis, then, are the sons and the brothers and the grandsons of victims, along with that very small handful of boys *and* girls both of whose parents happen to harbor the spondylitis gene.

For such target individuals it is a matter of no small consequence that ankylosing spondylitis does not usually interfere seriously with one's way of life, *provided treatment is started early*. This last phrase makes such obvious sense as to constitute a cliché; but, for a very simple reason, it should not be passed off lightly by anyone with a gambling-sized chance of developing the disorder. Most cases of ankylosing spondylitis, about 80 percent of them, have a way of getting off to a rather puttering start. They do not begin with the kind of fanfare that would prompt a 3:00 A.M. call to the family doctor, or even the making of an appointment for some Tuesday after next. To complicate matters, very early cases are occasionally easy to overlook, particularly if the symptoms happen to mimic those garden-variety backaches with which doctors' offices abound. If even so little as a casual "by the way," is dropped to indicate one's mother's father, for example, had "something-ankylitis in his spine," the entire diagnostic machinery might be set on a completely different tack.

Now usually spondylitis begins sometime between the ages of seventeen and twenty-five, only on occasion delaying its appearance till the thirties or the forties. Given a back problem of any kind in the high risk group, even the youngster in his early teens, therefore, deserves investigation.

Fortunately, the earliest signs of the disease are easy to detect: a simple X ray of the sacro-iliac joints will usually be revealing. Here, for some unknown reason, the disease most often leaves its introductory clues, sometimes long before the individual himself has felt a twinge of discomfort.

It would be misleading to say that such a young man's problems can be ended there. There is yet no permanent cure for this disease, but there is a most heartening gap between the state of his problem with the early institution of care and the state of his problem without it.

Fortunately, the treatment is neither onerous nor fraught with side-effects. There are more unpalatable medicines, for example, than nine or ten hours in bed each night and steady adherence to a healthy, nourishing diet. And while the special exercises prescribed for ankylosing spondylitis are critically designed to help prevent deformity of the spine, probably few of us

would be any worse, in terms of downright physical
fitness, by observing some of the same calisthenic
ritual. And, finally, there are the anti-pain and anti-
inflammatory drugs which can always be prescribed,
when needed, to comfort the man and calm the temper
of his disease.

When all is said and done, if the man with ankylosing spondylitis can keep atop his disease enough
to perceive it as a now-and-then stiffness and a now-and-
then ache, he will have achieved pretty much the same
distinction as so many of the rest of us who arise every
morning with the same complaint.

And, most certainly, he will be a far cry from that
pathetic prisoner of yesteryear who first taught surely
more than one small child—unknowingly and in the
span of briefest observations—compassion for man and
awesome respect for the forces that shape him.

GOUT

From the human viewpoint, gout is one of the most
ancient maladies. Its inclusion in the earliest medical
literature implies that it was already well known by
the time man had come by the art of writing and began
to use it to satisfy his compulsion to record for posterity
all things about himself.

From the evolutionary standpoint, however, gout
is a recent innovation—going back no further than an
event that seems to have been part and parcel of the
immediate prelude to man and his primate peers.

To understand this malady then, to appreciate
the hows and whys of this highly chronicled disorder,

one must look to a rather consequential mutation that lies buried now like a piece of broken pottery under so many layers of time.

It must have been one of those days when the hand of the potter shook, so to speak. When nature fumbled, that is, as she does now and then and—in the very instant of its recreation—dropped and shattered to bits the clay of a most crucial kind of gene, causing echoes that could be heard into the future and very possibly giving evolution, for a time at least, all the appearances of a revolution instead.

For in losing this gene, pre-man forfeited one of his own metabolic tools—a lively little chemical that had passed heaven-only-knows how many evolutionary tests—the little enzyme, *uricase.*

Now uricase, dedicated as it is to destroying the uric acid which the body constantly makes, is a rather indispensable commodity. For under uricase's catalytic hand, this relatively toxic substance, uric acid, is broken down into simple, harmless substances.

Obviously, then, the mutation presented its host —as it does his three billion some descendents today— with a problem of some immediacy. One that left him with no choice but to compromise the situation in any way he could and hope for the best.

Fortunately—thanks to primate luck and to a few allies from the bacterial sector—he managed to hurdle the crisis.

At least part of the uric acid now threatening to accumulate to critical levels in his body could, as things turned out, be broken down inside his gut by the bacteria ever present there. And as for the uric acid remaining? One can only conclude that having got this far on evolution's high sea, having dealt with navigational emergencies before, this pre-man creature wasted no time in resorting to that last-ditch measure: jettison.

Not that he was able to bail enough of it overboard at any one time—to excrete enough of it, that is, through his kidneys and into his urine—to keep himself completely *free* of uric acid. But he could and did dispose of sufficient quantities in this fashion to keep himself out of trouble, as do his three billion descendants, incidentally, even today. And so the story might end there with no one the worse for the nautical scare and no such thing as gout haunting the ship's log were it not for the fact that some people simply tend to make *more* uric acid than others, or to excrete *less* of it, or both. The net result, of course, is a somewhat higher body level of uric acid in some people than in others. And even then no mention of gout might ever have been made were it not for the fact that in *some* of these latter, and a minority at that, the excess uric acid tends to precipitate out in tiny crystals in the joints. And it is this sort of happening that does *not* escape mention in the ship's log—to say nothing of its mention by the owner of the joint.

For this is gouty arthritis.

In all fairness, gout is hardly the fault of uricase, of course—or rather the *lack* of uricase. The tendency to make too much uric acid or to excrete too little is caused by another kind of gene that has nothing to do with uricase. All the same, had man not abandoned uricase, or vice versa, he would still have the wherewithal to handle whatever excessive amounts of uric acid any of his other genes might be inclined to produce. If the blueprint for uricase had not got itself so unceremoniously lost in the deep dust of the millennia, gout would not exist.

And, very possibly, neither might knowledgeable man, sapient man. But more of that story in a minute.

Now the gene that makes for excessive uric acid is far from being identified and comfortably cataloged to everyone's satisfaction. It is not even clear if the responsible culprit is a single gene or a gene team, or even if the genetic factor is necessarily identical in every case. The very fact that excess uric acid is due to over-production in some people and to under-elimination in others does seem to suggest that not all such instances—and therefore not all gout—are one and the same condition. That genes of one sort or another do indeed play a heavy role in the genesis of the defect, though, seems relatively certain.

Due to hormonal differences, perhaps, women seem to be able to carry such gene or genes without effect. At least instances of excess uric acid or arthritic attacks prior to menopause are rare. Even though symptom-free, however, women carriers are prevented not one iota from transmitting the trait to their sons.

Excess uric acid, then, and its inheritance, is of concern primarily to men.

If he has a father or brother with the uric acid defect, with or without arthritis, a male's chance of developing a similar defect may run as high as one out of two.

Now certainly not all of the men who inherit the

trait are headed for trouble. Nearly a third of them, however, after the age of thirty, will indeed experience attacks of gouty arthritis. And a fifth of those who do —plus a few of those who do not—will have the occasional bout of kidney stones as well.

Rarely, the odds are even greater.

For a somewhat elusive reason, the sons of gouty mothers seem to be particularly prone to arthritic events, as are those men whose parents *both* possess the uric acid defect. That a greater arthritic risk is portended by two affected parents than by one is not surprising, perhaps, in view of the powers inherent in double-barreled inheritance.

All in all, harmless as the defect most commonly is, its potential for trouble is still high enough to justify a few simple precautions on the basis of nothing more than being a male with a close blood relative—grand-parent, parent, or sibling—known to have either the uric acid defect or overt gout.

As an example, let us take the case of the pre-adolescent son of a man with gouty arthritis. Because of his age, whether or not he shares his father's defect, his uric acid level is likely to be low. By the time he is sixteen, however, it will have begun to climb, mainly because this is the sort of thing that normally occurs in sixteen-year-old boys. If, thereafter, the amount of uric acid in his blood is average for his age, and a simple blood test can quickly determine that, his chance of having escaped the defect is good. In fact, the older he gets with nothing but normal test results, the better his chances would seem to be.

If on the other hand he *has* inherited his father's

propensity for making uric acid, then sooner or later
—and very possibly in his late teens—his blood will
begin to show an amount of uric acid which is excessive for his age. Now there is a strong feeling among
rheumatologists that such a lad—or anyone else for
that matter, regardless of age, who is none the worse for
his uric acid excess—probably needs no treatment beyond avoiding those certain well-known provokers of
the gouty attack: joint injuries, unnecessary stress, and
over-indulgence in food and alcoholic drinks.

Such measures are not necessarily a guarantee
against arthritis, of course, but they help. And when
they do not prevent it, they may at least reduce the
severity and the frequency of attacks.

One could argue here that the example is all well
and good for the boy in question because his father
was *known* to have gout—tipped his son off, in effect,
by developing arthritis. But what about the boy whose
father's excess uric acid maintains an uninformative
silence? Fortunately, today, he does not often have to
wait for the sudden midnight anguish of a close kin
to alert him. The test for uric acid is becoming almost
as routine a part of physical examinations as the test
for hemoglobin, reducing the chance that his father's
defect will never be detected.

A second and obvious advantage in knowing that
the defect is present, of course, is the opportunity,
when and if symptoms *do* appear, for immediate diagnosis and treatment. All too often the symptoms of
gout do not begin in the typical way—with that ex-
plosive onset of a painful joint in the dead of night
that leaves no one hard put to guess the trouble.

The man forewarned whose symptoms begin, say, as a vague, aching stiffness in the legs is far more likely to get himself an early diagnosis than the man not similarly armed with the knowledge of being at risk. And the earlier his diagnosis, it follows, the sooner his treatment and the more *manageable* his disorder. This is not to say that treatment does not help the man with long-standing gouty arthritis, but it cannot undo the permanent trademarks left on joint and kidney tissues by previous attacks.

If there is one disease the rheumatologists like to crow about it is gout. And for good reason. Short of permanently curing the disease—which, like any other inherited defect of metabolism, would require some tricky engineering at the level of the genes—rheumatologists have come up with a scheme for its near complete control. There are drugs used to suppress the over-production of uric acid, thereby eliminating one source of the problem; there are drugs used to increase its elimination, thereby hitting at another; and there are drugs used to take the pain and the inflammation out of angry joints in a fashion that has been described, even in the stodgy language of medical dissertations, as "dramatic."

In final effect, therefore, the man who knows he is at risk and, even so, chooses not to seek help in the earliest stages of gout is doing himself a bit of an injustice.

In the last analysis, moreover, he is even making mock of the very compensation nature may have made to him in return for giving him gout. But to understand why that is so we must go back now to a piece of broken pottery deep in the dust of the millennia, to a fossil gene, to the very beginning of the story of gout.

To leave off discussing this disorder with no mention of its eccentricities would constitute a negligence of sorts. Such eccentricities, for example, as its predilection for the well-shod and the well-indulged, its rarity in African nationals contrasted with its common occurrence in American Negroes, and its notorious prevalence in certain population groups, like Filipino men and the Maoris of New Zealand. Good living, sex, and even ethnic group—each seems to provide gout with a basis for bias.

Eccentricities such as these are actually tangent to the real climax in the story of gout, of course, having only to do with the nitty-gritty of hormones, genes, and ways of life. The real climax, in an evolutionary sense, lies in a bias of a very different sort—an unabashed preference on the part of gout for the brightsters among us.

It has not been by chance that when the rosters of the gouty have now and then been counted, the number of notables among them—like Isaac Newton, Benjamin Franklin, and Martin Luther, to name only a few —has often been enough to give the list a little of the aura of a "Who's Who." Moreover, when large groups of the gouty have been compared with the nongouty, the gouty groups have been found to average out with a slightly higher intelligence. And as if all this is not impressive enough, groups selected on the basis of nothing more than excess uric acid tend to show the same thing. This is not to imply that a dullard cannot develop gout, of course, and that a genius has any recourse *but* to develop gout. Far from it, as a matter of fact. After all, we are dealing with averages only, and with whole groups, groups that must be fairly large before the small but significant differences between them in life achievement and intelligence become validly apparent.

The real significance, however, is not in the difference between such groups at all, which over the long haul is just so much nitty-gritty like the rest. The significance rather is in the association itself of uric acid with intelligence. An association, it has been suggested, that may possibly be a *cause-and-effect* affair. For if uric acid acts as a stimulant to the growing embryo's brain, as has likewise been suggested, it is entirely conceivable that the human intellect was given a launching pad of revolutionary dimensions that fumble-finger day that nature left some primate ancestor of ours without a gene for uricase.

And gout? Well, if gout is indeed the price a few individuals must pay for the state of intelligence of the species as a whole, then in all fairness it would have to be conceded that nature—though she left us with a problem, true—also gave us, in that same fell stroke, the nascent gift to solve it.

IV

Disorders of Vision

IN THE DEEP of the ocean, where no light penetrates, there lives a fish that has no eyes.

By evolutionary choice.

In the perpetual darkness of his habitat he has no need for them.

Within the reaches of the sun, however, just as Erasmus intimated, First-Eye in the land of the primeval blind without a doubt was king.

However crude a shadow-perceiving device the original eye may have been, it must have given its possessor a powerful if not altogether sporting edge over the sightless others of his kind, allowing its owner's sighted progeny to replace the older version of the species in record generational time.

And that must have been only the beginning.

Each set of mutations that improved on the design —that added devices for perceiving texture and color and depth, for example—must have been given its host species another evolutionary boost.

It is not surprising, then, that in the brief history of living time almost every animal species has developed an eye so elaborate that even Darwin, granted he knew nothing about genes, was hard put to explain it.

In fact, it is probably safe to say that complex forms of life could never have evolved at all without the prior advent of a piece of visual equipment, for the eye favored more than just the survival of its host. In ways we can only surmise, its very presence must have altered the stage on which nature continually auditions a species' genes. To an extent we can only guess, it must have lent respectability to at least a few mutations that—for lack of relevance in a creature unendowed with eyes—would otherwise have failed the audition.

Granted it took more qualities than a complex eye to shape the human line—or so one must conclude, for the eyes of many a lower form of life are equally complex. Still, a human being is no less dependent than any other animal on an ability to see. If anything, his dependency is greater than theirs, in view of the multitude of human needs that vision serves.

It is true, of course, that unlike other animals, a man can survive without sight. But it is also true that he can do so only in the company of other human beings. For an animal, moreover, survival *is* life. For man survival is only existence.

To live, *really* live, to experience life fully, man must satisfy a ladder of needs. And survival is only the lowest rung. Man also needs, if for no other reason than the fact that he can satisfy such needs, a sense of security; the pleasure of social belonging; a buoyant belief, founded or not, in his own significance; and, last but not least, the consummate satisfaction of self-expression—self-actualization, as that psychologist said who first described the ladder.

Now the significance of all this is that man, like it or not, cannot draw upon the physical environment alone to satisfy these needs.

That was the agreement he made, in fact, for the right of access to the path of human beginning. The terms he agreed to in a contract drawn up a million years ago, written in blood, so to speak, binding on all his heirs, and signed by himself with the flourish of a broken rock—

—with the first deliberate wielding of that first primordial tool—

—a broken rock no sooner seized with preconceived intent than it became a thing dynamic in itself. Became the foundation stone of a quasi-living structure —*culture*—that could no more be undone, once started, than that preman wielder of the rock could have, had he opted out, retreated into the instinct-ridden darkness of his evolutionary past. A quasi-living structure, built of the hardware and the software of man's own making—his tools, his values, his institutions, his ways of life. An environment of culture that at once became far more efficient, far more nimble in the picking and the choosing of human genes than the hand of *natural* selection.

Take that broken rock.

As surely as this first crude tool selected its most genetically gifted users for species perpetuity—by favoring the survival of those, for example, with the sharpest wits—such individuals, in increasing numbers, used those wits to institutionalize a good thing. To reinforce the tool, that is, as a cultural form. To improve on its design and application.

And as surely as man improved the tool, such improvements enhanced even further the selection of those whose special talents were to become the stock in trade of modern sapient man.

Man and his culture, then, evolved together, each deriving from the other through an extravaganza of positive feedback relationships. Each is therefore totally dependent on the other.

Without his natural environment, true, man could not survive. But it is only in contact with his cultural creations—those stepping-stones of his genetic progress stretching out into a sea whose opposite shore has only that reality that he himself will give it—that man, *as man,* survives. That he expresses his full potential. Satisfies, as it were, that ladder of uniquely human needs.

Culture, like man himself, is derived, then, from an animal history that could never have been written in the absence of an eye.

Thus to the past, the present is often inescapably committed.

On the premise of vision, even now, our cultures are created and the means for their transmission to our progeny designed. Our arenas of living—from the highway to the classroom, from the work-a-day office to the theatre to sports—are all narrowly conceived of within the limits of our unconscious, visual bias.

In the land of culture, small wonder, then, if he without sight feels at times like evolution's stepchild.

It is equally unsurprising that some of the most voluminous contributions to our knowledge of medical genetics, concerned as it is with genes that in any way infringe on man's evolutionary rights, have been made by those who specialize in the care of the eye. As a result, the rogues' gallery of miscreant genes known to commit one or another kind of crime against the eye now contains no less than 250 well identified faces.

For a single organ, this is an impressive number of offenders. And it is a reflection, in part, of the fact that the eye is no simple device but an intricacy of interrelated parts, each the product of a multitude of genes.

In view of its complexity, the marvel may be that nondefective eyes exist at all, that the vast majority of hereditary defects are rare, and that the truly common ones—described below—are so amenable to treatment.

CATARACT

As a clouding of the lens, cataract does to one's image of the world what a dirty thumb print on a camera lens does to a finished photo.

Now the offending thumb may belong to any one of a number of different culprits, many of which, like an injury or German measles in the unborn child, carry no hereditary clout.

Moreover, many a cataract that *is* genetically induced is inherited not as cataract *per se* but as part and parcel of some broad disorder whose signs and symptoms characteristically go far beyond the eye.

A certain proportion of cases, however—the bulk, perhaps—are due to genes whose resulting defect is a solo flaw in an otherwise normal person.

Of these defects, the most common, the so-called "senile" cataract, earns its genetic label primarily from the fact that variation in the rate of aging is itself genetically determined. Thus, while almost everyone by the age of sixty has some degree of clouding of the lenses, in certain families "senile" cataract seems particularly prone to an early onset or a rapid course.

Unfortunately, nothing can prevent a cataract from developing, even one that is due to genes which manifest most typically in adolescence. What *is* subject to prevention is the permanent loss of sight. If and when a cataract progresses to the point of interfering with one's ability to function, it can simply be removed.

As a general rule, then, there is little headstart to be gained from knowing, before the fact of cataract itself, that one may be at risk.

There is one outstanding exception to that rule, however. Whatever cataract lacks for urgency in anyone else, it makes up for with a vengeance in the infant.

Certain of nature's timetables, it seems, are immutably fixed. One such program is her schedule for instructions, that tutelage in the everyday art of seeing that she offers only to the very, very young. For seeing *is* an art—not the automatic outcome of a pair of eyes but a *skill*—one to be learned by the very young brain in that most impressionable period of its earliest development or not at all.

Much past the age of one, the child who has not yet mastered that art likely never will, as would be the case, for example, if at the very time he could have been, should have been learning, the world was hidden from his view by heavy cataractous curtains.

Now infantile cataract of the inherited sort is almost always due to a gene which fails to express itself in only one out of twenty who host it and whose receipt from a single parent is enough to produce the disorder.

Since infantile cataract, if not present at birth, wastes little time thereafter in developing, the chance of its occurrence is of concern primarily to affected parents of infants who are new, prospective, or potential. Given one such affected parent, each offspring's chance of cataract is 50 percent, reduced in reality to 45 percent by that 5 percent chance he might carry the gene without showing it.

Should *both* parents be affected, an offspring's chance of coming out unscathed is 25 percent, and if he *is* affected, there is one chance out of three that he carries the gene not in a single but in a double dose— one gene from each of his parents. Though his defect would not necessarily be any the worse for that redundancy, his someday-offspring will have lost whatever chance they might have had to escape the cataractous gene.

Now infantile cataract is not common enough that couples with both members affected should be any more than a rarity. And indeed they would not be, were it not for the match-making hands of human practice and perception. For mating is rarely as random, nor love as blind, as is generally supposed. Geniuses, for example, rarely marry persons who are mentally deficient. People with strongly opposing religious views are less likely to mate than those with views more comfortably compatible. And the fact of it is, the visually handicapped tend to marry each other far more often than would be the case if all matings were a purely random affair.

Moreover, some of the very mechanisms man designs to compensate the blind, such as special, segregated schools and camps, often inadvertently aid and abet the hand of mating bias. And anything that fosters intermarriage among the visually handicapped fosters also the chance of intermarriage of persons whose handicap is due to the same genetic defect.

A far more common situation of course, is that in which one of two normal parents is from an affected family. If the gene for infantile cataract compensates at all for its indomitable nature, it does so to couples like this. For its presence is 95 percent unlikely in anyone with normal eyes. In the offspring of such a couple, then, the chance of cataract is only 1 percent.

Now a final and crucial word. While infantile cataract nearly always affects both eyes, it is by no means an all-or-nothing proposition. And though, like the waterfall from whence it got its name, it may involve enough of each lens to shut out all but the light of day, it often affects so small an area of the lens that its host is never aware it is there. Moreover, its appearance in any one family is remarkably consistent. The defect in an infant, then, is likely to be no more nor less severe than it is in the affected others in his family.

Any infant born to a parent known to be affected, however mildly, should nevertheless be given the benefit of the doubt by having his eyes examined shortly after birth and periodically thereafter for at least a year.

In the case of cataracts severe enough to call for an operation, an infant's only chance for useful vision may well depend on surgery's being done sometime during those evanescent weeks in which the chance of surgical success, increasing steadily as the cataract matures, intersects his ever-*decreasing* chance to learn to see.

If the cataracts are not severe, periodic observation to be sure they are not getting worse may be all that is required. So long as an infant is using his eyes, he is learning to see. In such mild cases, a physician may simply wait until the child is old enough to voice his own complaint—in the absence of which there may be little point in treatment.

Finally, if repeated examinations throughout infancy fail to reveal the semblance of a smudge on the lens of either of an infant's eyes, in all likelihood infantile cataract never will develop. For there was that 50 percent chance from the outset that he would fail to inherit the defective gene.

It would be misleading to imply that the treatment of infantile cataract leaves a child with perfect vision. It does not. There is yet no way to remove a cataract without sacrificing the lens. And the lenses of a pair of glasses never substitute perfectly for the living thing.

Treatment, provided it comes in time, can, however, endow a child with sight.

Useful sight.

With a workable view of a world shaped and colored and set into motion by the dictates of human need. And like everyone else, with a right—no, a definite obligation—to share in its creation.

CROSSED EYES

It is prevalence as much as patency that makes crossed eyes, or squint, so generally familiar. Among school children alone at least 1 percent are known to be affected.

More impressive, if less apparent, is the fact that half of these children have permanently lost the sight of one eye. And that that forfeiture was made, ironically enough, for the sake of better vision.

It is enough of a trick for the brain to reconcile, or fuse, the separate images referred to it from *normal* eyes. When, as in squint, the eyes do not fix and track together, fusion is out of the question. The eyes must simply compete with each other for the attention of the brain—a state of affairs no less confusing than hearing the sounds of a different conversation in each ear.

One can always alternate his attention, of course. But, as is usually true in squint, if one eye provides him with a sharper image, he is very likely to give it his undivided attention by suppressing his perception of the image from the other eye exactly in the way one learns to use a one-eyepiece microscope while keeping both eyes open.

Now such disuse, if it becomes a way of life, does not augur well for the disregarded eye. Unheeded, that eye seems to lose heart, little by little to give up trying until it is no longer able, even if called upon, to communicate its passive mirroring of the outside world. Such loss of sight in an eye equipped to see is called *amblyopia.*

Squint itself is due to a defect not of the eye but of the muscles that control its movement.

Certain cases—those primarily in which the problem is muscle paralysis—are due to injury or infection. But, where the problem is lack of proper balance between muscle push and pull, as most cases are, it is heredity that seems to play the major contributing role. Thus, on an average, 10 percent of the siblings of affected children are also found to have squint. This figure rises to 17 percent if a parent is also affected.

Precisely *how* the genes exert their influence, though, is still an amiable bone of professional contention.

Is squint the direct result of a refractive error like farsightedness? Or is lack of muscle balance inherited as a defect in itself which more often than not depends on a co-existing error in refraction to manifest itself? That most such errors do *not* result in squint, and that some cases of squint, particularly outward squint, occur in the absence of errors in refraction, would seem to suggest that the latter explanation is more valid.

Either way, the answer is probably academic. For either way the prevention of squint, in the majority of potential cases, lies in the early correction of one or another of the following errors of refraction.

FARSIGHTEDNESS

The inability to see near objects clearly is by far the most common refractive error in children. Unlike its counterpart in those over forty, its presence in children has more to do with the size of the eye than with the aging of the lens.

Hyperopia, as the professionals call it, shows a definite predilection for the children of parents who were similarly affected.

To put all cases down to the same genetic cause would be nonsense, however, for hyperopia can result from any one of a number of different errors in one's refractive equipment. It is difficult, therefore, to garner much more from the data on hand than the fact of hyperopia's obvious familial bent—and of the greater heritability, oddly enough, of its milder forms.

Suffice it to say, then, that a history of childhood hyperopia in either a mother or father implies enough of a risk to any of their offspring to warrant early investigative action. Since the defect is usually present at birth, examination then or any time thereafter should reveal it.

Oftener than not, the defect will be minor enough that the child will not require eyeglasses. If required, glasses are generally all that he will need.

Lest the simplicity of that treatment deceive one as to its significance, let him consider for a moment what it means to the child. Not only will glasses, if needed, provide him with a view of his most intimate world, that one that lies within his touch, but very possibly—if he had any tendency at all to squint, and squint indeed prefers the hyperopic child—they will safeguard his right to two-eyed sight.

NEARSIGHTEDNESS

The opposite of hyperopia is myopia or nearsightedness, the inevitable result of an eye that is too long. Like hyperopia, myopia defies a simple, single genetic explanation.

In some families the defects acts like a dominant trait, cropping up in every generation. In others it limits its appearance to one generation only. Rarely, it is even more selective, preferring to appear in the sons of mothers who carry the trait without effect themselves. Such diversity, of course, is merely the sign that those genes that govern the dimensions of the eye are legion.

It is safe to assume, then, that any child in whose immediate family myopia exists would seem to be a likely candidate for that affliction.

Unlike hyperopia, myopia is a long time coming on—at least as childhood is measured—for the first detectable signs, as a rule, do not develop until the child is in school, often so caught up in the pressing protocol of the educational process that he may fail to notice how far the blackboard has receded, how blurred to deception are those chalky symbols—those chalky stepping stones of his individual progress, as it were—until someone else discerns the fact that he is struggling too hard.

Moreover—since he may not be aware of how much he has missed, never having learned it to begin with—whatever holes he has accumulated in the fabric of his knowledge may not be easy to mend.

There is a second danger in delayed detection. While squint is more common in the farsighted child, it can and does occur in the myopic child, too. Moreover, as is true in hyperopia, to postpone action until visible signs of squint appear is dangerous, for amblyopia may claim the sight of the weaker eye before the squint is marked enough to make any cosmetic difference.

The child born into a family with myopia, then, should be vision-tested not only in early childhood but periodically throughout his school years. And such checkups should be carried out even in the absence of complaint, for children are less inclined to complaining than they are to making-do.

Except for a very severe, progressive form that is more nearly a degenerative disease of the eye than a simple error of refraction, myopia is easy to control. Glasses, changed as indicated by changes in the error, are all that most myopic children need.

Mixed Errors of Refraction

Clean categories are a figment of human invention. Nature patently abhors them. On some individuals, she confers a far greater degree of myopia than she does on others. She shows the same disdain for categorical rigidity in the degrees of hyperopia she parcels out.

It is only to be expected, then, that occasionally a myopic eye finds itself teamed up with a hyperopic

mate, or a slightly hyperopic eye with one extremely
so, or a normal eye with a mate having either error.
Anisometropia it is called—a significant difference in
refraction between the two eyes.

Now anisometropia, itself, seems to run in families. While its existence in a parent or a sibling calls
for the same kind of action as does myopia or hyperopia
alone, it flags a special warning.

Even if his error does not interfere with vision,
the child with anisometropia can get into serious
trouble. Take, for example, the child with marked
hyperopia in one eye and only mild hyperopia or normal vision in the other. Since his markedly hyperopic
eye is handicapped only for close range vision, he will
generally see well with both eyes, but not at the *same
time*. When the image in one is sharp, that in the other
is fuzzy.

As a consequence, he tends to alternate their use.
Now this eye, now that. It is not binocular vision—not
three-dimensional sight—but it works. Unfortunately,
though, since it does deprive him of the opportunity to
use both eyes at once, anisometropia subjects him to the
same danger that attends the child with squint. Should
he show a consistent preference for either eye, sooner
or later he will forfeit the sight of the other.

Glasses are often all such children need. For
reasons of optical perversity, though, anisometropia is
sometimes trickier to treat than hyperopia or myopia
alone. And the results of treatment are not always so
dramatic. Even so, the sooner the defect is detected and
treated, the better one's chance of maintaining two-eyed
sight.

ASTIGMATISM

The ability to see clearly only a part of what it is that one is looking at often shows up in the offspring of anyone who is likewise astigmatic. Whether or not astigmatism is due to the action of a single dominant gene, as has been claimed, is a matter of speculation, for it behaves in only a sometimes-dominant way. Which is simply to say that in certain families, it is as likely to skip as to hit a given generation.

For any offspring of an astigmatic parent, then, the risk of astigmatism, on an average, is somewhat less than 50 percent.

Only when astigmatism interferes with comfort or vision are glasses needed, and glasses are all that are needed.

Since the outlook is excellent, and serious side effects are ordinarily no problem, the only reason for discussing astigmatism here as a disorder subject to some facet of prevention is a bit of recent evidence suggesting that the vision of the astigmatic, in his later life, may be slightly better, sharper all around, if he is given the benefit of glasses in his early years.

GLAUCOMA

From the inside of a tunnel on a foggy day the world is a pale gray disc suspended in the darkness. A grossly shrunken universe, more provocative for what it conceals than reveals, textured with half-images, suggestive only.

But one has only to run to the tunnel's mouth,

then, to dispel the illusion, to be at one again with the infinite universe of sight and light.

It is, after all—that view from a tunnel—a momentary distortion.

For most of us.

Not all. For a few of us—too many—it is the only reality left, that remnant of sight, that knothole in the darkness, so typical of well-advanced glaucoma.

In effect a glaucomatous eye is one which contains more fluid, *aqueous humor,* than it was ever designed to hold. A situation resulting when, because of defective plumbing, less fluid leaves the eye than is being produced. In such an event, of course, the resultant increase in internal pressure, unless relieved, may permanently damage the delicate machinery of the eye.

Such a situation can proceed at any pace, from one extreme of tempo to the other. If the onset is rapid, the eye—caught by surprise, as it were—has little time to adapt. It can only signal its distress in ways at once communicated to its host—as severe pain radiating so diffusely that its origin may seem to be a tooth or one's whole head, instead.

If the onset is slow—so slow that the eye adapts not only to the pressure but, exceeding its limits there, to the insidious loss of sight—there may be no signal at all. Indeed, the damage to vision may be so surreptitious that the darkness of the tunnel permanently obliterates the edges of one's sight before he himself is conscious of the loss.

Glaucoma commonly results as a side-effect of injury, infection, or diabetes.

A significant proportion of the balance of cases,

however, occurs on hereditary grounds. And the responsible gene is usually one of a distinctly dominant nature, sooner or later expressing itself in 80 percent of its hosts.

Since hereditary glaucoma is a disease of later life, the 20 percent in whom the gene stays silent are very possibly those whose affliction was scheduled for some date handily distal to the usual life span. Or again it may be that, in certain individuals, the nonglaucomatous partner gene is not as totally submissive to the desire of a mate with glaucomatous intent.

While the presence of the disease in a parent, then, confers on an offspring a 50 percent chance of inheriting the gene, there is only a 40 percent chance that he will actually develop glaucoma. If he *does* inherit the gene, of course, its failure to express would make it no less available to the next generation.

Given siblings affected, as well as a parent, one's risk of glaucoma is, in most cases, still 40 percent, for the disease in the sibling is simply a reflection of the parent's own disease.

Glaucoma only in siblings again connotes a 40 percent risk, or so it is safest to assume in the absence of an obviously nonhereditary cause. The apparent absence of the disease in parents is a dubious hook on which to hang one's chance of escaping the affliction.

If *both* parents are affected, the chance that an offspring carries the gene is 75 percent, and one-third of those who do inherit it will carry the gene in double dose.

If the closest relative affected with hereditary glaucoma is a grandparent, aunt, or uncle, one's chance of affliction dwindles to 7 percent—a risk still four times greater than that in the population at large.

The earliest detectable signs of glaucoma tend not to appear until after age thirty-five—after which the frequency of the disease mounts steadily in carriers of the gene. Periodic examination, then, of close blood relatives—siblings, offspring, and parents, too—of anyone with hereditary glaucoma should begin no later than the age of thirty-five, or even thirty, and continue throughout life.

For anyone at a risk as high as 40 percent, the simple test offered in mass-screening programs is not adequate, for that test misses too many early cases of glaucoma. A combination of special tests is generally recommended instead. But the pay-off, when and if glaucoma does develop, can be tremendous, because the sight one has at the time that treatment is started he generally retains.

Treatment itself may amount to nothing more than a daily ritual of instilling drops in both one's eyes, though to be successful this ritual must be adhered to for the rest of one's life. Where drops alone are not enough to control the disease, surgery generally will.

Provided treatment is started early, then, the outlook in glaucoma is good.

It is only recently the case. At least as time is measured in the myopic purview of man, for the disease did not lack for recognition in the distant past. "Blue-gray" the ancients called it—even as we do today, borrowing from the Greek, *glaucoma,* meaning "color of the sea."

Color of the eyes turns to agate in the finale of the disease. That final stage at which sight is reduced to total blindness.

Not to darkness. Not to blackness. Only to the nothingness that one perceives through eyes, like those of the back of the head, that are not there.

Within the reaches of our contemporary sun— out on that stepping stone where man, en route to whatever destiny, now stands—there is absolutely no excuse for such a plight.

V

The Anemias

IN SUCH MYRIAD disguises does nature gain her access
to the current inventory of a species' genes—where, in
the interests of its further evolution, she tampers with
pricetags at the counters of its heritage—that she is
only rarely caught in the act.

Let one look about him for her evidence, for she
is at work now, in one disguise or another.

Looking, one cannot tell. All things appear as
usual. Nothing at all suspicious on the scene—unless—

Unless perhaps that recent upset in the weather?

Or that sea of high rise dwellings? But *whom* does
she favor in that disguise? And *how?*

Or might those be her stealthy fingers one glimpses
now in the slinking pall of contaminated air poulticing
the city?

One cannot tell. One can only suspect everything
now, not knowing.

Her disguises are too good.

Still, history is littered with the discards of her past masquerades, with bits of her evidence, after the fact.

The hoary whiteness of an extinct glacier sifting through the aggregate of prehuman genes for skill and providence was surely nature after all.

And that fractured rock, the first tool—how cleverly in the hand that wielded it was her own disguised.

So she comes on.

Now as a glacier—now as a tool—

—now as a mosquito, winging buoyant in the all-concealing darkness of a jungle night, in search of blood—

Nature—incognito—come again to manipulate the inventory of a population's genes, to alter the odds with which long-time favorites vie for majority status with their own mutational forms.

Thus, through her subtle touch, does a rare mutant gene occasionally rise to evolutionary eminence, to a prevalence that marks it as a common, if not predominant, characteristic of a population group. But for only as long, of course, as nature's preference persists. Should she change her mind, what was an asset may become a species' cross to bear.

It is, after all, the risk a species runs for the privilege of making evolutionary peace with a changing environment.

How many of man's more common genetic maladies achieved their prevalence in just such a fashion is a matter of speculation.

That *some* of them did, however, is a matter of fact.

The evidence is there. It lingers still in the populations of contemporary man. And nowhere is it quite so blatant as it is in the case of the inherited anemias. Specifically, those two conditions whose "anemia" label stems from their association with red blood cell destruction—and whose tens of millions of carriers around the world far outnumber those of any other anemia with a hereditary bent.

One defect, *sickle-cell anemia,* is so called for the contortions into which it throws the red cells of its victim. The other, for want of a reasonable label, is named after the red blood cell ingredient in which the flaw occurs: *glucose-6-phosphate-dehydrogenase deficiency.* An ungainly name, but there it is. That is all there is. So, like the biochemists themselves, we resort to shortcuts and call it G6PD.

Fair enough. While so common a disorder should by rights have a common name, the truth of it is, as we shall see later, it was only twenty, thirty years ago that G6PD deficiency, rank as it long had been in human populations, took on the nature of a problem.

SICKLE-CELL ANEMIA

It is no complicated piece of art, the hemoglobin molecule—more like a child's toy, a ball gaudy with the color of iron and garnished with beads. Four long strings, roughly one hundred and forty beads in each, one hundred and forty amino acids strung together, one by one, in a ritual of order: *leucine, valine, cystine*

. . . named like chorus girls, on whose proper line-up hangs the outcome of the show, of the job to be done.

A conveyor of sorts is the hemoglobin molecule, being the body's oxygen-bearer from the lungs to the cells' metabolic hearths. A ceaseless, vital job, for the cells are ever-demanding. Let he who doubts it hold his breath for a minute or two to be convinced.

If the job is ceaseless and vital, though, it is, in all frankness, also a little bit dull. Sufficiently so to make one wonder at the tenacity with which the molecule holds to the given order of its cast.

If so many chorus girls deep, a single substitute face appears—a single amino acid bead is replaced by another—who should care?

Who would notice?

Out of all the audience in that vast theater of human habitat, who would notice so miniscule a change?

Strangely enough, someone does.

Too often one does notice.

Like that child lifting his head from the mat in a darkened hut in Mozambique—*he* has noticed—that three-year-old hunching forward in the corner there, doubled over on the mat, fragile fingers gripping the swollen abdomen now as if to pluck out the pain.

Under his mother's palm his forehead burns. He has not wept for hours. Only pants between his screams, staring at the doorway. There, where the sun when it bursts will catch on the leaves of the acacia and set a hundred broken shadows to dancing on his bed, it is still dark. The sun, his mother says, will ease the pain.

Across the room, his sister, Wiyata, sleeps. Eight,

she is, and robust as a lioness. *How hard he breathes!* How long is the night! "The sun," she repeats, "will take away the pain. We shall go the river tomorrow to watch the boats, you and Wiyata and I—"

How long is the night!

How different is the act—even the darkness then does not conceal it. The *child* has noticed. Tonight he has—and how many times before? How many painful crises before this final one tonight?

It does not matter.

Not now, an eternal vigilance later, for the night is done.

He does not notice the pain. That, or the sun bursting into the doorway now, gently to cover him with the trembling shadows of acacia leaves.

Nor does his mother notice, still beside him, eyes closed, counting.

Of three children only Wiyata now, pressed against her, weeping.

Robust as a lioness. And now, in the thought of her daughter's vigor, the mother finds some small comfort. As if the fragility of the others were somehow compensated for in this one. Even as she thinks it, unaware that she is toying with the secret of one of nature's most ironic tricks. That the grave in which she lays her son is in reality the sacrificial altar at which certain threatened populations, for eons, have paid with their few for the survival of their many.

But that is jumping ahead of the story now. Ahead of nature itself.

For it was nature, of course, lurking back-stage all along. Nature who directed the substitution to begin with—through a mutation of the gene whose job it is to string those beads together—and in so doing converted the normal hemoglobin molecule into one with grossly deviant behavior.

Called hemoglobin "S" for the sickle-shaped spasm into which it can throw its red cell hosts, this deviant molecule differs from the normal hemoglobin "A" so slightly that its chemical identification, a few years back, made scientific headlines. Yet so radically different is it in another way that its detection in the blood has long been a prosaically simple task. Deprived ever so slightly of oxygen, the cells that contain this hemoglobin "S" will all appear, through the eye of a microscope, as small, red, crescent moons.

And that is the heart of the problem—the ease with which sickling occurs. For it is the shape and stickiness of sickled cells that account for their clogging the capillary vessels and, hence, for their own destruction. In those who harbor a double dose of the mutant gene, these episodes of sickling translate as painful crises, severe anemia, and early death.

It is a pair of sickling genes, then—one from each of one's parents—that results in lethal disease. Lethal enough to claim the lives of 80,000 infants every year.

Not in Mozambique nor Africa alone do these deaths occur. It is not on the basis of race that the altar exacts its toll. Graveyards as far away as Greece, Israel, and Turkey give mute testimony to that fact.

It is rather the fantastic prevalence of the disease in equatorial Africa that gives this population its high-risk reputation. For in tropical Africa alone, one out of every hundred infants succumbs to this disease. And for every infant who does, there are twenty more who carry the gene in single dose, a far less disastrous condition known as the *sickle-cell trait.*

Within certain nations in that equatorial belt, in fact, the frequency of carriers of the single gene runs as high as 40 percent. And their North and South American descendents have not gone completely unscathed, for even in the United States, one out of every ten to eleven Negroes is a carrier of the gene—of the sickle-cell trait—with the result that *sickle-cell disease* is one of the most common chronic disorders of American Negro children.

Now the sickle-cell trait has long been considered harmless. While its host makes hemoglobin S, he also makes sufficient hemoglobin A to keep him out of trouble, at least in the run of the mill situation.

On occasion, though—oftener, perhaps, as new technology introduces new environmental hazards—problems do arise. Extremes of the same situations that provoke a crisis in the child with sickle-cell disease—that lower the supply of oxygen to any part of the body—can produce clogged capillaries in the carrier of the traits as well, causing pain and permanent tissue damage. Moreover, there is evidence that the pregnant female with the trait is especially prone to infections of the urinary system.

Though rarely, the carrier state can even result in sudden death, as it did recently in four young military recruits undergoing strenuous physical training at an altitude of 4,000 feet. Totally unexpected, their deaths served at once to put the sickle-cell trait into a new and sobering perspective.

From the estimated four hundred single-gene carriers undergoing similar training at that base—only an estimate, granted, for the army does not routinely test for the sickle-cell trait—it would appear that under those given conditions of altitude and physical stress, one out of every hundred carriers of the trait suffers the self-same fate as the individual with sickle-cell disease.

In its own way, then, the inheritance of the sickle-cell trait is no less important than that of the disease. It is far more prevalent than the disease; it is not invulnerable; and it is totally amenable to the simplest preventive measures.

The risk of inheritance, moreover—for both disease and trait—is easy to determine, for the genetic basis is fully understood and the causative gene, when present, can always be detected.

Thus, given one parent normal and the other with the trait, each and every offspring has a fifty-fifty chance of being, likewise, either normal or a carrier of the trait. None will have sickle-cell disease.

If both parents carry the sickle-cell trait, the chance that a pregnancy will result in a normal infant is 25 percent. The chance is 50 percent that the infant will have the trait and 25 percent that he will have sickle-cell disease.

Take a practical example, the usual one in which the diagnosis of sickling disease in the infant of apparently normal parents comes as a complete surprise to everyone. In such cases, the above risks hold for all their future children, since their affected child is sufficient to identify them both as carriers of the trait.

Should the child with sickle-cell disease survive long enough to procreate—and with the best of treatment many of them do—he has no option but to pass along the sickle gene to any offspring he may have. If the other parent is normal, none of their children will have the disease but all of them will be carriers of the single gene. If the other parent carries a single gene, each of their children will, with equal probability, have either the trait or sickle-cell disease.

Should both parents be affected with sickle disease—granted the rarity of such an event—so will every one of their offspring.

Now detection of both the trait and the disease is inexpensive and simple. Moreover, rapid screening tests exist which make it possible to survey populations en masse.

However the carrier of the trait is detected, though, as a casual participant in a population survey or the concerned and conscientous relative of someone known to be affected, the same precautions hold. And by and large they all boil down to pretty much the same thing: the avoidance of any situation known to curtail one's oxygen supply—like mountain-climbing or other excessive exertion at higher elevations, traveling in aircraft that is not fully pressurized, underwater swimming, prolonged exposure to the cold, tight fitting garments and alcohol intoxication.

For the pregnant carrier of the trait, early and continuous prenatal care should help to make for the early recognition and treatment of any infection in the urinary system that happens to develop.

Unfortunately, the child with sickle-cell disease

has no such easy out. True, in the United States affected children not uncommonly survive into adulthood. But that lone case who attained the age of forty-eight—though a source of medical pride—is a medical record still. Nor is living, even with the best of modern treatment, without its woes—either for the child plagued with crises or the problem-plagued adult that he might someday live to be.

So he manages now and then to cheat death's altar for awhile. For some extra years of grace to leave a share of his comfort there in place of life.

It is an improvement.

But the reminder is no less there. And one wonders —knowing nature does not allow a felonous gene such prevalence unless someone profits vastly in the process —what was the gain? And how was it achieved?

How? Only listen.

Listen to the sounds of the past, in the static of the millennia, for that one distinctive note—

Listen, even now—today—in the evening air of Mozambique—along the verdant trails of Cameroon, at the sloughy edge, come dusk, of an Arabian oasis— listen—

There you will hear it. Coming out of the night. The high-pitched drone, sustained. The soft but penetrating sound of the mosquito—there, winging in the darkness—hungering for blood.

Miniscule creature—bearing a creature even more miniscule than itself: the parasite of malaria.

Look to the malarial belts of the world for the clue. For malaria was the great cartographer who mapped the territories of hemoglobin S.

Look to the child grieving with her mother in a hut in Mozambique—to the 40 percent of her compatriots who share with her the sickle-cell trait—for it is they who have reaped the profit. Spared sickle-cell disease by virtue of their hemoglobin A. Spared the more lethal effects of malarial assault, oddly enough, by virtue of their hemoglobin S.

Hybrid vigor, it is called. And the sickle-cell trait, by all admission, is the most remarkable example of such vigor known in man. In that critical period from infancy to the age of five there is no doubt that the child with the trait is less likely to die of malarial infection than the child who makes only normal hemoglobin A.

Little wonder, then, that the sickle gene has flourished so in populations given to doing battle with malaria. And that the most vigorous of such populations, as reflected in an ample prevalence of carriers of the single gene, are inevitably those with the greatest frequency of sickle-cell disease.

It is a story told before—for the survival of many, a few must die.

Still, it is a story without an end.

Even now there is a chapter being added in the western hemisphere, and another possibly being started back in the homelands of malaria.

Among American Negroes the carrier rate has suddenly begun to drop. One contemplates the most tempting of several possible explanations. Where no malaria exists, the carrier individual loses his advantage. Or, rather, the normal individual loses his *dis*advantage. More normal individuals surviving dilute the ranks and lower, as an arithmetic achievement, the percent of those with the trait. And the life expectancy of children with the disease has apparently not been lengthened sufficiently to have balanced the effect.

Whatever the reason, however, the decline is apparently real.

Meanwhile, in those homelands of malaria— where the draining of swamps and the liberal use of pesticides would eradicate not only the mosquito but the virtue of the sickling trait—something else is happening.

For mosquitoes, like men, are subject to genetic mutation. Let only an infinitesimal fraction of the mosquito population possess a mutant gene that makes them somehow pesticide-resistant, and in only a few short seasons their kind will predominate the species in the areas exposed.

So, it is happening already. Here and there, in old-time haunts where malaria had begun to wane, the disease shows signs of increasing again.

A wearisome, worrisome show.

What does one do?

Continue the endless search for new and different pesticides, each with its own potential for disruption?

Destroy the mosquito through methods more biologic?

Alter the malarial parasite itself to a form noninjurious to humans and hope for its competitive replacing of the harmful versions of its species?

A hundred possibilities. A potpourri of sober plans and wild thoughts. Not one of them—should it, could it, be effected—without the potential of causing unexpected and unwanted problems elsewhere in the system.

Still, regardless of possible problems, there are certain chances one must take.

So long as the mosquito haunts the night in Mozambique, man will try to negotiate for a better survival deal.

It is in his nature.

It is, after all, nature *in* man. But nature with a purpose now. Nature with a conscience.

For the truth of it is that that mindless creature is capable of either purpose or conscience only when she comes in the human disguise, only when she acts in the shape and substance—through the mind and the heart—of man himself.

G6PD DEFICIENCY

It is an old saying in Sardinia that he who eats the fava bean and then falls ill had best beware his taste.

The malady to which the caveat applies, however, is confined to so small a handful of population groups that elsewhere in the world it has never aroused much more than scientific sympathy.

Favism this ailment is called, a novel, if sometimes lethal, affliction reserved for a selected few whose strange sensitivity to the fava plant leads to red blood cell destruction, or *hemolysis*.

Hemolysis in favism is ordinarily so severe that it not only darkens the urine and yellows the skin but so greatly threatens the body's oxygen supply that, without transfusions, up to 10 percent of its victims die.

Only where the fava bean is found, however, does the malady occur. Under circumstances so ethnically exclusive, who could have recognized the malady as the patient herald of a someday global epidemic? Of a rash of outbreaks far beyond the pale of the fava bean —in Indo-Chinese swamps, in far-flung military bases, here and there in North and South America, among stay-at-homes who had never seen a fava bean, much less consumed one.

Above all, who could have known—when the epidemic was well upon us, twenty years ago—that the agent of its contagion was a mutant gene?

Now a gene is hardly contagious, of course—except as one may pick it up through that exposure to his parents that results in his conception. Moreover, its spread in the gene pool of a population is a time-consuming affair. No gene gains species eminence overnight, nor even in the span of a generation.

How then could one explain its epidemic-like behavior?

Quite simply—now, in retrospect.

The mutant gene had been prevalent for a long, long time in many populations. Except for its unpredictable run-ins with the fava bean, it had enjoyed an anonymity of sorts in return for good behavior. And likely it would have continued to, had someone, or something, not ruffled its disposition. For the gene appears to have a side effect which is definitely advantageous. Like the gene for hemoglobin S, it seems to confer on those who carry it a measure of protection against malaria's more lethal complications. In areas where malaria is prevalent, then, he who carries that gene is more likely than his noncarrier comrade to survive.

And so it is not by accident that it occurs—this gene for what we now call G6PD deficiency—in a full one-third of the people in certain areas of Sardinia and Greece, or a fourth of certain populations in Africa and Malaysia.

In Saudi Arabian oases, in parts of Israel, carriers of the gene comprise a whopping 65 percent of certain tribal groups.

Even in American Negroes the carrier rate is not inconsequential—13 percent. Higher even than the carrier rate among this group of the sickle-cell trait.

Like the normal gene, from which it long ago derived, the mutant gene directs the manufacture of a chemical—G6PD—that serves as a metabolic choreboy to the red cells of the blood. But the G6PD the mutant makes is slightly different chemically from that of the normal gene.

Now, who is to say which one of them is better so long as the job gets done? What matters it that the G6PD of the mutant gene is not so energetic so long as its energy is sufficient for the task? Is it not conceivable, even, that the "normal" one is slightly *hyper*active?

It is a general genetic rule, however, that the worth of a gene is determined by its situation. And that situation that gave the gene its sudden unsavory reputation—that ruffled its disposition, reduced it to a handicap—was provoked by man himself. Man—and a passel of good intentions.

For it was the wide-scale use of certain, well-intentioned drugs, beginning twenty, thirty years ago, that started the epidemic. Drugs, it so happens, which, like the fava bean, are more than the mutant form of G6PD can handle. Drugs which, even more consistently than the fava bean in fact, cause anything from mild hemolysis to frank hemolytic crisis.

Ironically enough, moreover, many of these drugs, being anti-malarial in nature, are used to prevent the very disease against which the mutant form of G6PD appears to offer some protection.

In far-flung military outposts, soldiers by the dozen tinged mysteriously yellow. In the resident populations of the malarial belt—wherever the drugs were used—the same strange outbreak of jaundice caused by the pigment spilled from broken cells.

It is, in fairness, only an off-and-on disease. In the absence of those agents that provoke hemolysis, its victim is no less healthy than anyone else.

One might liken him to the hay fever sufferer who has no complaints in the absence of pollen.

The ubiquitous pollens, of course, are difficult to elude. But often so are the offending drugs. For the list of such offenders is not limited to the anti-malarials alone. More than twenty-five others have already been identified—like certain anti-bacterials, certain sulfa drugs in particular, a few of the common pain relievers, and even vitamin K. A list which will almost surely increase as new drugs are developed.

Crimes against the red cells, moreover, may not be limited to medicinal offenders. A recent study indicates that in a lead-polluted atmosphere—a common characteristic of congested urban areas—the child with

G6PD deficiency accumulates in his blood a higher
level of that poison than does the nondeficient child.
The possible implications of such a finding, if further
studies confirm it, cannot be taken lightly.

The children involved in this study were Negro,
moreover. And the defect in Negroes tends to be less
severe than it does in whites—a reflection, merely, of
the fact that the mutant gene for G6PD occurs in more
than a single version. How much more lead might
accumulate in those with defects more severe no one
yet knows.

It is not surprising, then, that a one-time scientific
sympathy toward a rare event has become, today, an
active global concern.

Aided and abetted by still another salient fact.

In males, a single gene is all it takes to produce
the maximum effect. Every male carrier, therefore, is
a potential case, and is subject to hemolysis.

It is a phenomenon that has to do with the somewhat special way in which the defect is inherited.

Consider the human cell with its twenty-three
pairs of matching chromosomes—each pair a dual contribution from one's parents, each carrying its allotted
load of equally paired-up genes.

Consider next that certain chromosomal pair that
has to do with sex—whose single members come in
either of two versions: X or Y.

Now it is an X combined with an X that makes
a child a girl, an X combined with a Y that makes it
a boy.

And the difference is significant to more than the
perpetuation of the species. It means, for one thing,

that none of the genes on a father's X can harm—or favor—his son. Had the boy inherited that chromosome, he would, of course, have been a girl instead, for his mother has naught but X's to give.

Moreover, since the Y is a chromosomal dwarf with no known genes to its credit, whatever genes his mother's X bestows on him will all have full expression, including the one for G6PD, for the chromosome X is precisely where that gene resides.

A son can inherit the defect, then, only from his mother. If she carries a single mutant gene, his chance of G6PD deficiency is one out of two. If she carries the gene in double dose—one on either X—his chance hits the ceiling: 100 percent.

The inheritance situation is different for a girl. In the first place, she has twice as many X's as a boy, a situation which, were it left at that, would endow her with an X-ful of extra genes. But nature—in an egalitarian spirt, perhaps—made a token correction long ago when sex was still an experiment in mammalian evolution.

Early in the life of an unborn female, one X or the other in each of her cells falls into a deep and permanent sleep from which nothing can arouse it. Like Sleeping Beauty, alive and well, with no Prince Charming to restore it.

Now which X suffers oblivion is a cellular decision, because each of two adjacent cells may boast a different Sleeping Beauty. It is a purely random affair with the rather mosaic result that, on an average, in half of a female's cells her father's X holds sway, in the other half, her mother's.

So it is even with such notorious X-borne genes as those for color-blindness and hemophilia. One can only assume—since these disorders occur in girls only when both X's are affected—that the activity of the normal X-containing cells is always sufficient to prevent the disease.

All the same the micro-evidence is there. With one fine test or another, one can usually find evidence of a mutant X-borne gene—as a diminished perception of color too slight, ordinarily, to be noticed by the female carrier of color-blindness; as a subtle but harmless prolongation of the time it takes the hemophilia-carrier's blood to clot; as a level of G6PD activity, in women carriers of G6PD deficiency, that is neither grossly deficient nor yet quite up to snuff.

Now should a woman carry a double dose of the mutant gene for G6PD, one on either X chromosome, she is as fully subject to hemolysis as any male with the trait. Moreover, since the mutant gene for G6PD is exceedingly common—in certain populations being less an exception than a rule—affected women are not uncommonly encountered.

For a daughter, then, the chance of G6PD deficiency is a more variable affair.

Given an affected father and a normal mother, 100 percent of daughters will be carriers of the gene, in a single dose, and therefore only mildly affected, if at all, by the hemolytic drugs.

Given a normal father and a carrier mother, a girl's chance of carrying a single mutant gene is 50 percent or 100 percent—depending on whether her mother carries the gene in single or double dose. In any case, she cannot be fully affected. The normal X which she acquired from her father assures her of that.

Only if both her parents are carriers can she be as affected as a male. And the chance that she will be— again depending on her mother—is either 50 or 100 percent.

Now, fortunately, one need not wait for an adverse encounter with a drug to make his diagnosis. Speedy, reliable tests have recently been developed which detect even the female carrier of a single gene.

It goes without saying, of course, that the blood relatives, including newborn offspring, of persons known to be G6PD deficient are top priority candidates for such testing—along with anyone who has had a hemolytic reaction to a medication of any kind.

Such tests have even been recommended, on a mass survey basis, for entire populations where the frequency of the mutant gene is known to be high.

So it is, after eons in the meritorius service of its species, that a gene sometimes finds itself reclassified as an evolutionary burden.

Certainly, he with the mutant gene for G6PD, given his choice, would opt to be without it.

One less precaution for him to observe, one less care to keep in mind—who would blame him?

Still—would the inventory of the species' genes not lose a little of its variety were the mutant gene to disappear?

When a species is threatened, does its chance of survival, after all, often not depend on its carrying in that vast bag of its collective genes a mutation to fit the occasion?

Should the carrier of the abnormal gene for G6PD be tempted to disparage it then, let him be reminded that as a bit of insurance in behalf of the species a mutant gene can only be collected on as long as someone carries it.

He may be living testimony to that truth.

For had one of his distant forebears not harbored the gene, he himself—given the untimely malarial death of a single ancestor in the life-line intervening —would never have come to be.

VI

Mental Illness

OUT OF THE luminescent tumbleweed of yellow dust, from the color of music and the voices of light, the Lord Himself takes substance now, coming ever more clearly into view until the chamber is suffused with the compassion of His presence.

Here, in the chamber's darkness, that vision comes to a Kiowa Indian waiting now to witness it—with his own eyes alone—that he might see himself a greater truth.

A vision—wrought by the substance peyote. The downy cactus in whose flesh a million dormant dreams lie awaiting the experience of whosoever should believe its power.

Peyote. Maker of dreams. Like certain drugs of man's own manufacture—amphetamine, and methamphetamine, and LSD—no less provocative of sights and sounds that do not exist than the forces of conventional madness. Than those internal agents that are given to evoking uninvited visions in the 1½ percent of all human beings who are mentally ill with either of the two major types of psychosis—schizophrenia and manic-depressive disease.

It was that eerie similarity, in fact—that mimicry by drugs of the symptoms of mental illness—that jolted scientists from a complacency born of having gone too long without a clue.

The effects of small doses of methamphetamine, for example, are often indistinguishable from mild schizophrenia. The effects of larger doses, over long enough periods of time, are often so like those of schizophrenia in its full-blown form—hallucinations and delusions, extremes of agitation and anxiety—that unless a patient is known to have been on drugs, it may be only his recovery, on being off them, that makes the diagnosis.

Moreover, evidence indicates that such reactions are not due simply to the activation of a dormant schizophrenia in those who are predisposed but are due solely to the drug.

For the scientists, of course, the finding was hardly just a clue. It was vastly more. However complex the cause of mental illness, however obscured by ignorance and myth, its duplication by a simple drug had to be regarded as a breakthrough.

It was a finding whose pursuit may yet result in the longest truthward step that has been taken since the very last witch or demon, centuries ago, was exorcised from the victim of untoward visions, and he was at last credited with simply being ill.

If certain drugs can produce a picture in their users which in anyone else would constitute an out-and-out psychosis—and it is this that gives the finding impact—might those with out-and-out psychoses, through some internal bent, be the victims of drugs of their own metabolic making?

Consider for a moment the potential of as commonplace a hormone as adrenalin.

Now adrenalin is the body's shock absorber, so to speak. It is the drug the body makes as its own built-in response to immediate stress. How would one who lost his temper fare if stalwart adrenalin were not there to toll at his heart and jack up his respirations to fit the occasion? Who knows? Without adrenalin he might simply collapse. Without that extra reservoir of strength that adrenalin saves for emergency situations —that surplus of energy one never knows he has until he needs it most—how would the caveman, in an unexpected confrontation with a tiger, say, have had the strength to run as fast as we have every vicarious right to believe that he did? In truth, the only misconduct of which one might accuse adrenalin is over-dedication— particularly in a world in which threats are, increasingly, of a sort one cannot meet with overt physical exertion.

All and all adrenalin, then, is a rather model hormone, one whose shapely plumpness, as organic molecules go, is not at all uncommon.

Should one try to touch it up a bit—through some biochemical sleight of hand add a few decorations, say a bangle of atoms here and there—who would fail to recognize the plump familiar form? Certainly not the biochemist—though neither, of course, would he miss those added touches. Nor fail to identify it now no longer as adrenalin but something very much like mescaline instead.

Mescaline. Maker of dreams. The active substance in peyote.

So, it is at least a cause for thought. Something, a possibility, one takes note of.

Could psychosis, by any chance, be due to a broken link in that metabolic chain of events that leads to the production of adrenalin-like compounds in the body? Who knows? One keeps an open mind to other possibilities, continues to query.

Somewhere, in one hypothesis or another, the truth is waiting. One has only to find it. And should those hypotheses that are already being pursued prove barren—well, it is the luck of well done research that it always yields something. For information, by definition, is never a void—even a finding which does death to a cherished idea. And the explosion of a hypothesis often shows up, if not in the increased strength of its rivals, in the birth of even more substantial ideas.

However hypothetic the cause of psychosis may be —however elusive is the discovery of the process by which it is produced—there is, at least, no longer any doubt that one of its ingredients is genetic.

That is a point deserving of special note because the evidence that establishes this fact has been either badly ignored or subjected to a third-degree unparalleled in any other disorder.

Why the apparent resistance to what the evidence shows?

Some of it undoubtedly springs from the still too widespread notion that what is gene-inspired man cannot undo. Granted he has yet to develop the know-how to perform anything such as a "genectomy," so to speak, to remove from one's cells whatever gene it is one does not want as deftly as a surgeon takes out one's appendix. But there is a tremendous leeway for therapeutic action between a gene's activities, confined as they are to the cell, and their final translation at the whole man level. And the myriad genetic disorders for which successful therapy exists—diabetes, gout, glaucoma, to name only a few—are testimony to that fact.

In part, perhaps, the resistance is a normal reaction to evidence that knocks at the props of cherished and honored beliefs. The subject of mental illness, of course, abounds with such beliefs, since hard data—quantifiable facts—are so difficult to come by in the abstract area of human behavior. Without facts, one must do precisely what the biochemists are doing now in behalf of the same disorders: hypothesize. If one cherishes a hypothesis, it is only natural that he feel some remorse at its subsequent disproof. Remorse that even certain biochemists will experience, too, for going as such scientists are, and should be, in several different directions, they cannot *all* be right.

And then there is that other tendency—the memory of which, as much as anything, may account for the resistance—to think of things as *either-or*. That is, as either genetic in causation, on the one hand, or environmental on the other. Granted, it is a misconception on its way out. But there is a hint of it still—or so it could be construed—in any implication that one or the other, genes or the environment, is the more important. Taken literally, the implication is absurd—much like stating that the one dimension of a rectangle is more important to its area than is the other.

What is really meant by such an implication, of course, is this: given the gene necessary for trait X, the probability that the environment, with its inherent variations, will actually allow trait X to develop is greater—or less—than half. Only that. If it were 70 percent, for example, then only 30 percent of those with the gene would be kept, by environmental vagary, from developing the trait. Should one infer, however, that the author of such a study meant to imply that the gene was therefore a good deal more important than the environment, one might quite understandably resist— particularly if he feared that those crucial features of the environment that are also required might somehow be lost sight of in future therapeutic shuffles.

Misconceptions, then, and choice of words are probably as much to blame as anything else for the delay in accepting what the accumulated evidence of forty years now confirms beyond any reasonable dispute: that, given the necessary environmental provocation, the development of schizophrenia or manic-depressive psychosis requires the presence of certain genes.

MANIC-DEPRESSIVE PSYCHOSIS

It is loss of contact with reality that distinguishes the victim of psychosis from those whose behavior labels them as either normal or neurotic.

What distinguishes manic-depressive psychosis from other kinds of psychosis is its victim's tendency to mood extremes. To alternations between elation and despair. Between wild euphoric behavior and morose withdrawal accompanied by a sense of infinite despondency that no amount of reason can dispel, such cyclic bursts of seemingly irrelevant behavior coming on without apparent provocation—without external help —as if controlled by some internal metabolic clock.

It is estimated that manic-depressive psychosis affects one out of every two hundred people. But that figure may be low, for no one really knows how many cases show up only in suicide statistics.

Now it is a paradox of sorts that the most common disorders are those whose modes of inheritance are the least understood, and manic-depressive psychosis is no exception.

Theories abound. The simplest holds a single gene to be at fault, one that is dominant enough over the likes of its normal partner to produce the disorder in half of those who harbor it. Other theories favor the notion that depression without mania—and it is true that many of the victims of manic-depressive psychosis never experience those compensatory bouts of elation —is a separate genetic disorder. Or, if not a separate disorder, that an additional gene of some kind is needed to round out the picture.

Without a well identified mode in tow, one must glean then what he can about the risks to the close blood relatives of a victim from the past experience of other affected families.

Such studies indicate that where a parent is

affected, an offspring's chance of developing the same disorder at some time during his life is, on an average, 20 to 25 percent. The same risk applies to the brothers and sisters of a case.

When one of a pair of *identical* twins is affected, so is the other—sooner or later—in over 90 percent of such pairs.

If a grandparent, aunt, or uncle is the closest affected relative, one's chance, on an average, can be assumed to be a good deal less than 25 percent but somewhat greater than that ½ percent prevailing in the general population. Unfortunately the data are too meager to be more specific than that.

If manic-depressive psychosis is actually a mixture of disorders, or if unrelated genes can influence its appearance, the figures in the previous paragraphs, of course, could exaggerate—or understate—the risk in certain families.

Thus, in many families in which only one or two cases of manic-depressive psychosis have occurred, the risks may be lower than stated. Likewise, in families in which manic-depressive psychosis abounds, the risks may actually be greater. To whatever extent the risk is increased, however, so is the chance that the unaffected do not carry—and cannot pass on—the adverse gene or genes.

As yet no reliable means exists of predicting the appearance of the disease before the onset of symptoms. It is claimed, however, that certain personality tests can provide a clue even in the child, years before the disorder's usual onset in the middle of adulthood.

However that may be, simple awareness of an

over-average risk, in itself, goes a long, long way toward the recognition of symptoms that would ordinarily have been ignored or overlooked.

It is a recognition that sometimes makes the difference between life and death.

Far too often manic-depressive psychosis is a lethal disease. And far too often, death itself—sudden, unexpected and self-inflicted—in tragic retrospect makes the diagnosis.

It is no statistical accident that among blood relatives of affected persons the suicide rate is ten times greater than in the general population.

Survival is not the only concern. For everyone who dies, there are untold others who, sans benefit of diagnosis, continue to suffer those swales of infinite despair. And needlessly, today. With the introduction a decade or so ago of certain drugs—biochemical keys, as it were, that actually unlock the victim from his moods —manic-depressive psychosis became at last a highly treatable affair.

By the thousands, its victims now are living fully productive, fully creative lives—doing, as nearly as anyone can tell, precisely what they would have done had they never been affected.

These drugs are not a cure, of course. If discontinued, those cyclic moods will generally recur. But the drugs, by and large, do *control* the disease. For they accomplish, in a sense—if not so easily or quickly— what a good pair of glasses does for that forty-year-old who has come to believe that publishers are using smaller print. They restore the world and all things in it to a real—a meaningful—perspective.

SCHIZOPHRENIA

Any malady that affects one out of every hundred people as consistently as schizophrenia does—in all races and cultures—merits the status of at least a minor trademark of the species.

Moreover, the world's thirty-five million victims do not complete the picture. Like the iceberg, they are but the visible cap of an infrastructure of another hundred million whose signs and symptoms, falling short of out-and-out psychosis, are referred to simply as the *schizoid* trait. A trait, in other words, which is schizophrenia-*like*.

Now the schizoid trait is easier to describe than identify, for its symptoms consist of such nonspecific features as anti-social behavior, extreme suspiciousness, sullen sensitivity, unreasonable fears, and marked rigidity of thought.

Still, there is no doubt that the schizoid trait as an entity does exist. Also, the trait is far more frequently found in the families of schizophrenics than in families without that disease, including those with other kinds of mental abnormality. The predilection of the schizoid trait for the blood relatives of schizophrenic persons is so apparent, in fact, that it was reported by asylum physicians more than a century ago from casual observations they made on visiting days.

The major distinction, it is claimed, lies between normal and the schizoid trait—not between the schizoid trait and schizophrenia itself, for the only difference between these latter appears to be one of degree. To anyone who is less concerned with cause than with incapacity, however, that difference in degree may be the crucial one. For schizophrenia is that portion of the spectrum beyond whose shaggy separation from the schizoid trait reality is lost, orderly thinking breaks down, and hallucinations and delusions reign.

Unlike manic-depressive psychosis, schizophrenia tends to come on rather early in one's life, with somewhat of a preference for adolescence and the early thirties.

It has been said that schizophrenia also has a predilection for lower socio-economic levels. A peculiarity which, on closer inspection, appears to be a characteristic not of the disease but of the way in which man garners data. For schizophrenia is often so insidious in coming on that one's slipping performance, by the time of diagnosis, has resulted in a corresponding slip in economic status. If one looks at its starting point rather than at the ending place, schizophrenia's predilection for the so-called lower classes seems to disappear. If anything, there seems to be a possible predilection for the upper socio-economic levels.

Differences in body chemistry between the schizophrenic and the normal individual have also been reported. None of these findings, however, have yet been totally confirmed, including that of the presence of that substance in the blood of certain schizophrenics which reportedly reproduces the symptoms of psychosis on injection in normal volunteers. And the more recent finding of abnormal substances in sweat and urine as well.

How typical such substances are of schizophrenia

in general, and whether they are cause or effect or pure
coincidence, is currently under study.

Almost surely, though, a biochemical difference of
some kind does exist. For biochemistry is the language
of the genes.

That the genes do indeed play a role in the genesis
of schizophrenic disease has now been well established
by a host of findings, demonstrating among other
things—

—that blood relatives of schizophrenic individuals
have a greater than average frequency of the same
disorder.

—that the offspring of schizophrenic parents have
a greater than average frequency of that disease even
when they are permanently separated from their families at the time of birth and reared in foster homes.

—that being reared in a foster home has no definite
connection with schizophrenia, either, for there is no
undue frequency of the disease among the children of
nonschizophrenic parents who are also raised from
birth in foster homes.

—that it is no peculiarity in an unborn child's environment, imposed by schizophrenia in the mother,
that increases his risk, for the children of schizophrenic
fathers are as prone to the disease as those of schizophrenic mothers.

While such studies have left no doubt that genes
are an essential ingredient in the development of
schizophrenia, however, like Pandora they have un-
loosed a host of controversies over the *likes* of that
ingredient.

Is it, for example, a single gene of autocratic bent?

Or a willy-nilly fellow given to expression only in the company of an equally willy-nilly mate?

Or a hatful of genes, perhaps?

Or is schizophrenia a mixture of separate disorders each with its own genetic author?

The most popular theory currently is that the disease is due to a single gene. One that has the capacity to produce anything from severe schizophrenia to absolutely nothing at all, depending on the whims of the environment and the sideline influence of certain other genes.

However that may be, various studies indicate that, on an average, about 10 percent of the offspring of schizophrenic parents develop schizophrenia themselves, while another 30 percent manifest the schizoid trait.

The same prevalence obtains among brothers and sisters of a schizophrenic, though the frequency of schizophrenia climbs to 20 percent if the disease occurs in both a parent and a sibling.

When both parents are affected, roughly one-third of the offspring develop schizophrenia, too, and one-third more develop merely the schizoid trait.

Among the partners of schizophrenic identical twins, 45 percent are also schizophrenic, and another 40 to 45 percent have only the schizoid trait.

Given only a schizophrenic grandparent, aunt, or uncle, the frequency of schizophrenia plummets to something very close to that prevailing in the general population—roughly 1 percent.

The risk of psychosis among the offspring of parents with only the schizoid trait is not yet known, but the scanty data indicate it may be somewhat less than when a parent is frankly schizophrenic.

Now the figures above are subject to some individual variation, due in turn to variations in environment and in certain other features of one's genetic make-up. Stress, for example, tends to increase the likelihood of psychosis, though why and how it does so is still unclear. For reasons equally obscure, the siblings of those who are only mildly affected seem less liable to psychosis than the siblings of those whose schizophrenia is severe. Likewise, persons of stocky build seem somewhat less prone than do the lankier among us, and when they do develop schizophrenia, the stocky ones, as a rule, seem to handle it better. As do those, on an average, with better than average intelligence.

Although it is claimed that the individual who is truly schizophrenia-prone can be detected, even in childhood, by a combination of certain physical and behavioral tests, there is yet no single, simple technique that can make this distinction. Among offspring and siblings of schizophrenic persons, then, it is the presence of deviant or problem behavior, suggestive as it often is of the schizoid trait, that normally alerts one to the possibility of proneness to psychosis.

Or *should* alert one, at least. For the prone individual himself is often in need of treatment—psychotherapy or otherwise—which, without recognition of his problem, he may not get. It is no professional secret that occasionally a person with the schizoid trait suffers as much impairment as the frankly schizophrenic. It also happens that many a schizoid individual, short of that impairment, needs the kind of therapeutic help he all too often does not get when his problem goes by any other label.

Moreover, recognition of proneness allows for immediate diagnosis—and therefore the benefit of treatment undelayed—when and if psychosis does develop. Though schizophrenia is often given to a rather insidious start, time can be crucial. If not to the course of the disease itself, at least to the course of one's life, to the quality of his existence.

Recall, for example, that strange affinity that schizophrenia seems to have for the lower socio-economic classes. And ponder on how needless that social decline might have been had treatment come in time.

Consider those other problems, too, that commonly plague the schizophrenic in that limbo interval between the onset of his illness and the day that he is finally diagnosed: family disruption, broken ties, divorce, and alienation. Thus are his major sources of security all too often seen to crumble at the very time he needs security most.

And then there are those problems that often result from lack of behavioral discretion: violations of the law, perhaps; or alcoholism, chronic and severe—which incidentally, however it may poultice his emotional congestion, can also act to mask his symptoms and delay his diagnosis.

In short, it is more than contact with reality that is at stake. For reality, reestablished, may be slightly bitter fruit if in that limbo interval things of value have been permanently lost.

Things that early treatment might have saved. For

like manic-depressive psychosis, the major symptoms of schizophrenia, in the majority of patients, can now be controlled through the use of appropriate drugs.

In the last few years, medications have literally revolutionized the outlook in schizophrenic disease. For though their use does not resolve the totality of one's problem—leave him totally symptom-free—it has at least returned the bulk of present day victims to a meaningful place in society at large, there to cope and contribute in a most acceptable way.

And that, of course, is only the beginning.

For the recent crescendo with which the story of schizophrenia has suddenly begun to unfold fairly hums with anticipation of things to come. Of ever-improving treatment. Of a sometime cure. Of a day when all of the answers are finally in.

And those questions that now still haunt the nights of scientific endeavor will be sated then.

And we shall know then, precisely, not only the nature of that basic genetic flaw, but also how environmental forces acting on the outer man—in their final interpretation at the level of the cells—conspire with that flaw to drive a man mad.

A climactic understanding it will be. Like a jigsaw puzzle, like a psychedelic revelation pieced together through the years by such scientists as could perceive the truth, lying larval as a dormant dream awaiting one's experience, in the pages of asylum history, in monotonies of data—in bangles of atoms, in colored sounds—in tumbleweeds of luminescent dust.

VII

Rheumatic Fever

LET ONE SLEUTH for rheumatic fever's favored haunts and the finger of history, without hesitation, will direct him to the northern latitudes.

It has always been so—rheumatic fever's penchant for higher altitudes and cooler climes. And so it is not surprising that the focus of efforts against this disease by those in medicine and public health has shown a like geographic bias.

Those efforts have paid off.

In the United States, today's child is less than half as likely to develop this disease as he would have had he been born in 1920.

It is a far cry from eradication, of course. But no disease in human recollection has ever been totally extinguished, not even the plagues of yesteryear's most infamous epidemics.

The decline in rheumatic fever, in fact, has been

111

apparent for so long now that the health profession, in the midst of self-congratulation, has admitted to a twinge of queasiness about claiming all the credit. Among other things, it was noted that the first signs of decline began forty years *before* the introduction of specific treatment measures.

Still, it was generally agreed, treatment must have put an added weight on an already sagging curve. Certainly there was no denying that treatment had reduced both the frequency and the severity of rheumatic fever's complications.

Thus was a jubilant profession so preoccupied with the beginning demise of the disease in its traditionally northern haunts that it failed to notice, until recently, how common a sight the child with rheumatic fever had suddenly become in areas as geographically sacrosanct as Africa and Asia.

What has been won in the battle against rheumatic fever, then, is only a hemispheric achievement. In the so-called developing nations of the world, the disease is now on its way to becoming a major medical problem. One reminding us not only that the battle is far from over but that the winnings to date are ours to keep, and add to, only so long as we continue to respect those two strange bedfellows who act conjointly to produce rheumatic fever.

That partner with the more familiar face, of course, is the bacterium known as a streptococcus. It is he who plays the introductory role, most often as an infection of the throat, in the drama of rheumatic events.

As all good streptococci should, however, he or-

dinarily runs his course after several days and, with no
particular fanfare, disappears. For another few days
the patient feels good. Then, one to three weeks after
the onset of the infection, as a rule, any or all of rheumatic fever's various symptoms suddenly appear—
painful swelling of the joints, migratory in nature,
enough to limit mobility at times; fever; rash; and, on
occasion, those aimless, uncontrollable movements of
the arms and legs that in the old days went by the name
of "St. Vitus' dance."

By and large, however, this strange melange of
signs and symptoms is eventually given to disappearing
on its own. In a sense rheumatic fever, then, is a self-
limiting disease which would surely have been granted
no more rank in the roster of human afflictions than in-
fluenza, say, where it not for its tendency, now and
then, to do irreparable damage to the heart—a tendency which, in the past, has expressed itself often
enough to have left a full 1 percent of today's American
adults with chronic heart disease. Moreover, rheumatic
attacks tend to recur with each new streptococcal infection, and each recurrence kindles anew the risk of
heart involvement.

Now characteristically, rheumatic fever shuns the
infant under two. Its favorite target has always been
the child between five and fifteen years. Likewise, it
has a slight but definite preference for the female sex.

It is none of those things, however, that most dis-
tinguish the disease's reputation for overt discrimination.

Witness its pick-and-choosiness when a streptococcus dressed for epidemic battle invades a "con-

tained" population, say an army group, whose intra-population contact is so sustained and intimate that virtually everyone becomes infected who is not yet immune to that particular streptococcal strain. The very "containment" of this population, moreover, makes it possible to determine every one of those who do become infected.

With such a denominator, so to speak, what kind of a showing, numerator-wise, does rheumatic fever make? The fact of it is, for every one hundred persons infected, no more than three acquire the disease.

On the basis of what credentials, biologic or other-wise, do the ninety-seven escape?

For the answer to that we must look now to the streptococcus' partner-in-crime—to that particular gene that makes the final determination of who, in the denominator of all infected persons, will get rheu-matic fever.

An elusive kind of gene it is, for its biochemical assignment in the body is still obscure, rheumatic fever perhaps being only its tangential consequence.

As a matter of fact, it may not be *a* gene at all but rather a *group* of genes. No one really knows. Evidence so far garnered, though, seems to favor a pair of genes, a single gene from either parent. There is also the possi-bility that certain additional genes have a kibitzing effect. At any rate there is no doubt that rheumatic fever occurs far more often in some families than it does in others, even in identical environments.

If a parent has had the disease, for example, the chance that each offspring will acquire it too, even-tually, appears to be 10 percent—a risk thirty times greater than that experienced by the general school-aged population.

Moreover, rheumatic fever in any child of never-affected parents connotes the same risk, roughly one out of ten, for each of his brothers and sisters. Should one of the parents have been affected too, the chance is slightly greater: nearly one out of six. For the offspring of parents who have *both* been affected, the chance becomes greater than one out of two.

A cheap and simple test, of course, which would tell one precisely whether or not he is really predisposed would be a great help.

Unfortunately, we do not have even an expensive, complicated one—beyond waiting for an actual attack to make that distinction in retrospect.

The following precaution then is generally recommended, across the board, for *all* siblings and offspring of any individual known to have had rheumatic fever. And only with tongue in cheek can one exempt from this group those who are over fifteen. For the very factors responsible for the dramatic reduction in rheumatic fever's prevalence have also tended, for reasons we shall look at in a moment, to increase its risk among young adults. No longer is a first attack occurring in one's twenties anywhere nearly rare enough to be the professional conversation piece it was. Rather, it is a first attack at forty that today gets special mention.

Now the target of that precaution is the streptococcus itself. For the early treatment—or outright prevention—of streptococcal infection is still the one and only reliable means of preventing rheumatic fever.

Accordingly, that precaution consists of getting to

one's doctor, more or less straight away, in either of two events. One of them, of course, is a sore throat. And not necessarily a very bad one either, for rheumatic fever has been known to follow infections too slight to produce any symptoms. If a throat culture, made from that cotton-tipped stick with which the doctor swabs one's throat, is negative at this time, no treatment may be needed. On the other hand, the very sight of the throat, or the severity of the inflammation, may be enough to make a doctor decide in favor of treatment even before the results of the culture are in.

The second indication for seeking medical help is a sore throat in anyone *else* in the household if its cause is known to be streptococcal. In such a case, depending on the circumstances, a physician may not be content to use even the small-sized doses of anti-streptococcal drugs that are normally preventive, but—preferring to err on safety's side by assuming that exposure has already led to infection—he may opt for full treatment instead.

There is a precautionary postscript. Treatment, when prescribed, should be faithfully adhered to for the entire recommended time. And that word of warning from one's physician should not be taken lightly. For typically, streptococci tend to seek the sanctuary of those warm protective niches with which the throat abounds, and medication must be taken long enough to get the very last of the hangers-on.

Now it is true that rheumatic fever can often be prevented if treatment is started even as late as eight or nine days after the onset of infection. However, if

one has any option in the matter, there seems little to
be gained by calling it that close, for rheumatic fever
does not always observe that generous, one- to three-
week period of grace.

It is a testimony to the potential pay-off of such
precautions that rheumatic heart disease is now offi-
cially considered a *preventable* affair.

It is the *only* chronic heart disease as yet accorded
that distinction.

And that preventability, in no insignificant measure, applies even to the youngster who has already suffered his first rheumatic attack. For, oddly enough, the
very failure of prevention, or of its application, all but
guarantees that failure will not occur again.

Once a child has actually suffered a bout with
rheumatic fever, he is put on anti-streptococcal drugs
and kept on them, day in, day out, year after year, until
he is an adult. With *this* child one takes no chances at
all, for he has proved his vulnerability beyond the
shadow of a doubt.

That his first attack of rheumatic fever may have
left his heart undamaged is no guarantee that the second or third attack will do likewise. Moreover, if
damage *has* occurred, each subsequent bout adds further insult to his heart. To make matters worse, children with heart involvement seem to be particularly
prone to recurrent attacks.

Thanks to that ritual of daily medication, however, over 95 percent of its adherents never have a
second attack. And that is quite some change from the
days when the recurrence rate ran as high as 75 percent. Moreover, that 1 to 5 percent of today's crop of

children who do suffer further attacks includes a fair proportion of adolescents who "forget" their medication every now and then, like four days out of five.

The effect on rheumatic heart disease itself has been nearly as dramatic. Where roughly seven children out of ten, in days gone by, wound up with damaged hearts, only two or three out of ten today have any such residual effect.

The last remaining bastion of rheumatic fever, then, is by and large those first attacks, the vast majority of which are now within the pale of prevention.

And so, potentially at least, rheumatic fever would seem to be at last on the verge of hibernation. On the brink of that semi-dormant state sometimes alluded to as "conquered."

How long this hibernation lasts, however, once achieved, will depend on many things. For the waxings and wanings of this disease are determined, after all, as much by human behavior—human restlessness and aspiration—as they are by the power of "miracle" drugs.

Take its striking decline since the turn of the century, when the miracle drugs were no more than a wistful professional dream. And the cause of rheumatic fever was anybody's guess. If indeed anybody in those days could afford to dedicate much time to guesswork, having far more urgent, far more epidemic matters to attend to. Like improving levels of sanitation and implementing hygienic measures in order to control, for example, such more pressing problems of the day as massive streptococcal outbreaks. Far too busy, they were, in fact—spurred on by a rewarding decline in streptococcal disease—to credit an equally obvious, albeit enigmatic, decline in rheumatic fever as being anything but a most fortuitous fluke. Only in retrospect, some forty years later when the cause-and-effect relationship between the two diseases was quite incidentally discovered, was the puzzle finally solved.

Those same achievements in the control of streptococcal spread, of course, help to explain rheumatic fever's recently increasing tendency to appear in older children. With fewer streptococci being passed around, a child's chance of infection is decreased at any given time, thereby increasing the chance he'll reach adolescence or adulthood before being exposed to any strain of streptococcus. The widespread use of anti-bacterial drugs may, incidentally, be having the same effect.

And what of that surreptitious increase in rheumatic fever in the southern latitudes, in the warmer climes?

It coincides, of course, with the restless emergings of new, half-alien economies in the "still developing" areas of the world. It parallels the ingressions of technology, the crumbling of old life styles, the grafting of cultures, one on another.

True, some of that increase is almost surely deceptive, a reflection of more accurate diagnosis. The child with rheumatic fever in such areas today is far more likely than ever before to be correctly diagnosed and therefore counted in the tally.

By and large, however, the increase is real. For industry's promise of manna—and the élan of burgeoning cities—have been luring untold rural millions into a state of mobility and togetherness which, in favoring streptococcal spread, must more than overcome the handicap imposed on its communicability by plain hot weather. The standard of living, moreover, has not gone up enough to negate that effect.

Too often, in truth, the élan of the city is but a mirage, and reality turns out to be a crowded ghetto, unemployment, and a level of living vastly lower than that that was left behind.

Moreover, the phenomenal reduction in the rate of death among infants under one—for many a nation the only improvement in the standard of living that can be said to be outstanding—may actually be contributing to the rise in rheumatic fever. More and more infants who in past days would have died are now surviving into the ages at which they are most eligible for rheumatic fever's discriminatory draft.

It was not so different, once upon a time, in the countries of the north. And what one sees today, in the southern hemisphere, is probably only a rerun, then, of an old familiar story. A setting of a stage at which all civilizations sooner or later arrive—culture by culture —to bide some little while before moving on.

And the streptococcus itself? It still prefers—and likely always will—the higher altitudes and cooler climes that favor its survival. Given its druthers, it would also prefer those human hosts who suffer nothing on its account, for they too favor its survival.

But the truth of it is the streptococcus has, of late, had little to say in the matter. Other than the odd mutational ace it pulls from its sleeve, the cards that it plays are from a deck that man himself, increasingly, has stacked.

VIII

Epilepsy

THE FALLING SICKNESS, said the priests of ancient
Greece, is divined by the gods. He who cries without
warning and falls to the ground is suffering the puni-
tive wrath of the gods themselves.

High time, they said, that once and for all the
matter be considered solved, settled, closed.

And then one afternoon, in a fit of scientific pique,
Hippocrates sat down with pen in hand and took the
lot of them to task. The priests were simply drumming
up an alibi, he said, for having obviously failed to
cure the epileptic. A tactic, he reprimanded them, that
could bear little useful fruit, for to cure an affliction
one must first of all be honest about its cause.

The falling sickness, he informed them categori-
cally, was due not to gods nor demons at all but to
heredity.

Thus, in that blunt pronouncement 2,400 years

121

ago, did Hippocrates put his finger, if not on the complex weave of epilepsy's cause, at least on one of its most substantial threads.

That his claim was a little simplistic one must be willing to overlook. For in view of how little he had to go on in that pretechnologic age—in a culture that viewed the experimental methods of science as a vulgar substitute for contemplation—he achieved far more, relatively speaking, than most of us do today, *with* technology, *with* scientific knowhow.

Were he now alive, he would almost surely be a physician among physicians still.

But Hippocrates belongs to the past. And it is just as well, perhaps. To be where we are, we needed him there.

Nor could he, were one to bring him back, give a fair demonstration of his genius without the knowledge that we have today. Though that is a tantalizing thought to pursue all the same—rousing him from that longest night of all, rustling him out of that all too permanent bed to make, we beseech him, just four more calls. As diagnostician par excellence, to come with us to witness some maladies that perplex us even today.

To hurry with us up the darkened alleys of the past, out into the afternoon of a Sussex garden, say, where the woman with the graying hair sits upright on the chaise longue now, startled at the sudden staccato beating of her heart: "I really loathe it when it happens, these dreadful palpitations. Now they'll go on like this for three, four minutes, you know, until my feet are like ice and by that time I shall feel quite clammy all over."

Or across an ocean and a continent to that young man, there, at work, behind the cyclone fence of a California institution. He with the gentle, comely face. What would the master physician have to say about *him?* "Twice—would you believe it, man?—I tried to kill my brother. Come Monday I'll have been here seven months." So young he is. How old would Hippocrates guess? Surely people today look younger than they did, then, when the face of a young man might, by twenty-two, be pitted with pocks and too soon etched with the harshness of life. But this one, it is obvious, has all his years been loved and tended well. It is in his face. A kind of softness that pervades his expression, and one looking at him now is suddenly suspicious that in the liberating privacy of night he is still capable of boyish tears. "Wild. I was raging. 'I only asked you for the time,' my brother said. After. And they all kept wanting me to tell them why. 'What made you so mad?' But I couldn't remember. Man, would you believe it? I couldn't remember doing it."

Or take the master physician now to the fevered five-year-old in that farmhouse on the outskirts of Sydney. Let him search the little boy's throat for signs of inflammation, listen with an ear to the child's chest for the rasping sounds of pneumonia—and find nothing there. *Strange malady.* And there is a look of unmistakable perplexity now in those astute old eyes. "But he's been like this before," the child's mother says, and having said so seems somewhat consoled. "He'll have been just fine, then I can tell looking at him he's suddenly got a fever. Never a cough. Nor earache. Just the temperature. After a while he'll vomit and feel better and tomorrow I'll have a hard time keeping him in bed."

But now, for old times' sake, let us take Hippocrates back to his own old haunts. To Athens. Past it. Down toward the Sunium cape to where the blue-as-ever Aegean laps today at the feet of westernized apartments in the suburb of Glifada and the Greece-that-was is no more than a scattering of mementoes—here a broken bone of sculptured marble protruding through the turf—there a sequence of letters, ΓΛΥφΑΔΑ, *Glifada*—here and there, the striking blondness of an occasional child, like that one listening to her uncle now, from across the dining table—

Notice in particular, Hippocrates, how bright are her eyes. How alive her laugh. For surely, even as you watch, she will be suddenly consumed as if by infinite boredom that drains her face of light and fixes her empty stare upon her uncle's countenance—though, clearly, she hears nothing that he says.

What does the master physician have to say to that? What is his diagnosis? The child is a dreamer? Perhaps. For look at her now—as suddenly, in the instant, her laughing, live-eyed self again.

But no. No, this time you are wrong, Hippocrates. Though the question is hardly fair, for coming from the past you could not possibly know that what you have seen today—every bit of it—is as surely epilepsy as is the falling sickness itself. So stay for a moment and listen then. For these are the fruits of the seeds you yourself once sowed.

Surely now and then, in those Grecian evenings of your time, you must have watched the storm clouds gather over the sea, beyond Poseidon's bluff perhaps, and seen the thundering silver of Zeus' weapon hurled across the sky.

So, it happens also in the substance of the brain. In every miniscule cell a bit of that self-same energy from which the lightning bolt of Zeus was forged. For it is the nature of these cells to discharge such energy that they might communicate one with the other, and all together with the man himself.

Though they do not normally all communicate at once.

Should enough of them, like the thunderbolt, discharge at once, and again and again, from the center of the brain, the force of it will make a man fall mightily to the ground to foam at the mouth and fight as if with unseen gods or demons. But should a man be given to storm clouds in more peninsular regions of his brain, then he shall break into a rage instead and attack not unseen gods or demons but whatever man or woman should stand close by. And if the region of storms be in that substance of the brain that governs not a man's thoughts or his deeds but the rhythm of his organs, then fever shall flush him instead, or his heart shall convulse, or his head begin to ache as if the thunderbolt had truly come from the hand of Zeus.

But now a kind of circumspect excitement has begun to kindle in those sage old eyes—a questioning incredulity—"But if you know all these things," and his voice when it comes is like an echo spiraling upward through the well of time, "then is it not true you would that you could have done more?"

But only like an echo now, for the voice of course

was always one's own. Out of the well of consciousness, not of time. Hippocrates lies unmolested still. And the scene, from its beginning, was never more than an illusion of an illusion. One's own illusory survey of a situation from such a perspective as Hippocrates himself might have had, a taking stock—through someone else's eyes.

It is sometimes the *only* means of taking stock. To view the present, that is, not from its obscuring midst but from a site apart, the better to judge how far we have come. The better to know what it is that we have done, and what it is we have yet to do.

And what the voice of our insight, thus enlightened, tells us now cannot be denied. For it is true that we know many things where epilepsy is concerned and it is also true that, for what we know, there is more to do, and for what *cannot* be done, there is more to know.

In 2,400 years one might have hoped, if not for a permanent cure, at least for a fail-proof means of seizure control. Yet our growing repertoire of anti-convulsant drugs today does make it possible to keep 60 percent of cases seizure-free and to reduce the frequency of seizures sufficiently in another 25 percent to relieve them of their major handicap at least. Neither the priests, by comparison—nor Hippocrates either—had any success with treatment at all.

And the tally, per se, of epilepsy today—that estimated 1 to 6 percent of the population that suffer anywhere from one to multiple seizures—how does it compare with the tally in Hippocrates' own time? Surely those sundry infections which, unbeknownst to

Hippocrates, can leave one epileptic must have been rife in ancient populations.

Still, is an individual not more likely now than then to survive the infection—and therefore to experience that epileptic postscript?

But what of trauma, injuries to the head, as another notorious dealer of epileptic seizures? Was the past, the distant past, not brutally traumatic? Perhaps. But truly no more so than is the present. War, for example, was certainly no more prevalent then than now, nor were its weapons as traumatic. Moreover, the automobile had not yet been invented. And both war and cars are generous contributors to the cause of today's convulsive seizures.

Yet injuries such as those sustained before or during birth were surely more common in the past, for is it not true that modern obstetrical care has tremendously reduced the incidence of damaged infants?

Yes . . . . But also no. For when good obstetrical care results in infants who are normal rather than defective, it also unavoidably results in infants born defective who would otherwise not have survived.

And what of those contributions to the epileptic tally that are of a less environmental nature? Well, there is little doubt that that most consistent thread in epilepsy's complex weave of causes—the genetic one—has persisted through the centuries to appear as evident as ever in the contemporary epileptic scene. And that, in spite of the sanctioned genocidal practices of the last two, three millennia. Such customs, for example, as the immediate castration of any man who should be seen to convulse, and the instant burial sans benefit of death for the pregnant epileptic woman. Customs which persisted until only a couple of years ago—with the same intent, with the same illogic if with less ostensible brutality—in the form of laws forbidding the epileptic to marry. As attempts to "decontaminate" the gene pool of the species, or at least that part of the species privileged to live within the jurisdiction of so protective a body politic, they have failed rather badly.

It was destined from the outset that such attempts would fail. For at least half of all those individuals who are epileptic on genetic grounds unwittingly conceal their identity by never having a seizure. Moreover, a good share of those who are frankly epileptic convulse for reasons primarily nongenetic.

And it is well for all of us that those efforts have failed. If every individual who is here today by virtue of an epileptic forebear were suddenly to disappear, so—in that self same instant—would the species, lawmakers included.

It is doubtful, of course, that anyone in the past ever recognized how abundant in the human population are those genes with the capacity to make like Zeus, or how extremely varied is the nature of their storms. How gentle their genetic wrath compared with that of epilepsy's more environmental causes, such as those all too insoluble scars that sometimes follow injury and infection. Or how much easier genetic epilepsy is to placate, to subdue with simple medication, and how very much more likely to fold up tent in the night of adolescence—plagued as that night may be by other kinds of storms—and steal into ever-after silence.

The more purely genetic epilepsy is, in fact, the easier as a rule it is to control. And the better is its ultimate outcome.

And nowhere is that phenomenon more apparent than in the falling sickness itself, that most familiar of all epileptic convulsions: the *grand mal seizure*. The "large fit." The one which strikes an individual to the ground—there to cause him to foam at the mouth and fight as if with unseen demons—as a result of a thunderbolt originating in the center of the brain.

It is, in a sense, a paradox that disturbances of the central brain are also the source, sometimes in one and the same individual, of the most gentle of all epileptic seizures, the so called *petit mal* type, the "tiny fit."

The petit mal seizure is a most unobtrusive affair, consisting of brief loss of consciousness only. But though it is often so fleeting that a child, walking, may merely slacken his pace for a step or two, it is often so frequently recurrent that in the aggregate it deprives the child of sizeable chunks of his everyday. So perforates his consciousness that he has trouble making sense of the pieces of life he perceives in between.

Petit mal it was that drained the light from the eyes of the child in Gilfada and left her for that instant in suspended animation.

Now epilepsy of this central type—whether grand or petit mal or both—is more often than not genetically-inspired as a malady exclusively epileptic. Only 40 percent of such cases appear to be due entirely to nongenetic agents such as trauma, infection or tumor, or to inherited disorders in which seizures are only one of several, often more serious, problems.

In that 60 percent of "pure" epilepsy, so to speak, that occurs on genetic grounds, the basic defect —likely metabolic in nature—has yet to be clearly established.

Regardless of its nature, however, the presence of the defect can be readily detected. For in the pattern of the brain's electrical behavior—as shown in those test recordings known as *electroencephalograms,* or simply EEG's—epilepsy of the central type produces a peculiarity so exclusively its own, and so different from the pattern that normal persons show, as to give its presence more or less promptly away.

Moreover, the defect appears to be due to a single and rather dominant gene, for half the siblings and offspring of those whose epilepsy is of this central type show that same peculiarity in brain wave pattern. At least if their EEG's are taken at the proper time, for the peculiarity tends not to appear until the age of four or five nor to persist, in the majority of cases, past sixteen.

In itself this brain wave abnormality is harmless enough. It is rather the seizure with which its presence correlates that is the problem. And the truth of it is that only half of those with the abnormality ever experience seizures. Moreover, of those who do have seizures, many will have no more than one or two. What makes for the difference is still a matter of some speculation. Perhaps even in this highly inherited form of epilepsy, an environmental insult—however unproductive of seizures it might be in anyone else—is also required.

In actual figures, the risks seem to stack up something like this: given an affected parent or sibling, one's chance of having at least one seizure runs from 20 to 25 percent. There is only a 10 percent chance, however, that such a person will have more than two or three such attacks—and only a 5 percent chance that he will develop a severe and long-term epileptic problem.

If one's closest affected relative is a grandparent, aunt, or uncle his chance of having at least one seizure is roughly 5 percent while his chance of a severe epileptic problem, is not much greater than the risk of epilepsy in the population at large, perhaps no more than 2 percent.

Of all forms of epilepsy, hereditary seizures of this central type are generally the easiest to treat. Grand mal particularly is easy to control. And if petit mal is sometimes a little harder to suppress, it is even more inclined than grand mal to eventual disappearance. For petit mal seizures rarely if ever occur in adults.

In light of that tendency of the brain wave to revert to normal during adolescence, it is not surprising, of course, that inherited epilepsy of the grand mal-petit mal type is so given to disappearing.

Neither is it surprising that the risk of seizures among the close blood relatives of persons who develop grand mal epilepsy not as children but as adults is generally low, since proportionately more of such late-onset cases will have been caused by factors predominantly nongenetic.

The above risks, then, apply to a somewhat exclusive group which, in lieu of EEG confirmation, can best be said to consist of those whose seizures begin in childhood or early adolescence, take the form of grand or petit mal or both, and are not preceded by obvious injury or infection.

For other types of epilepsy, the risk situation is not at all clear—beyond the fact that heredity definitely plays a less imporant role.

Take, for example, the form of epilepsy characterized by so-called *temporal-lobe* or *psychomotor* seizures.

Here, the stormy disturbance occurs somewhat off-center, in or around one or the other side lobe of the brain. And the thunderbolt that emanates therefrom produces a storm that resembles neither the falling sickness or the gentle petit mal at all.

It is a convulsion, instead, of behavior and sensation. And though it comes in nearly as many sizes and shapes as the people it affects, in any one victim its picture is rather consistent.

Thus one individual may be gripped by sudden, uncontrollable panic, while another takes to repeating, like a broken record, whatever his activity or stream of conversation might have been at the time the seizure began. In other victims, the seizure may be a strange sensation instead, or an out-and-out hallucination or delusion which, except for the abruptness with which it starts and ends, may so resemble the symptoms of mental illness that its victim may be loathe to describe what he remembers having felt lest someone think him mad. And there are those, too, for whom a seizure is a sudden burst of rage, sometimes with violent behavior, like that described by the young man behind the cyclone fence in that California institution.

Psychomotor seizures may last for seconds, or hours, or days. Though consciousness is not necessarily lost, often only blunted, there is no real recollection afterward, or a hazy one at best, of what transpired in the attack.

In the majority of cases of psychomotor seizures, unlike epilepsy of the central type, injuries to the head and other nongenetic factors appear to be primarily to blame. And this, in part at least, may account for the fact that psychomotor epilepsy tends to be more difficult to control than grand or petit mal.

Even psychomotor seizures, however, are not totally immune to the influence of genes. Recent evidence now indicates that in at least a portion of all cases —perhaps nearly a third—a genetically determined predisposition exists.

On occasion, both psychomotor and grand mal seizures occur in the same individual. This situation, in any given instance, would seem to favor a primarily environmental cause. There is always the possibility, of course, that such an individual is epileptic on more than a single score, or that there are certain genes that increase their host's susceptibility to a *variety* of seizure forms.

It is in a state of enlightened confusion, then, our present day knowledge of epilepsy as a whole. For that reason it is difficult to say with any degree of precision just who is at how great a risk.

Even the EEG is not a great help in the matter. Granted, its normalcy in the five- to sixteen-year-old sibling of a child with grand or petit mal seizures can be most reassuring. And certainly a normal EEG in the close blood relative of any epileptic is more assuring than one that is grossly abnormal. In itself, though, such a normal EEG is no guarantee that seizures will not occur, for the EEG is not too effective in detecting stormy foci in the deeper reaches of the brain, relying as it customarily does on electrodes held against the outside surface of one's head.

In general, then, the safest assumption would seem to be that the siblings and offspring of anyone with epilepsy not clearly due to nongenetic forces have a somewhat greater than average chance of developing recurrent seizures severe enough to require long-term medication. That sweeping statement might well include the siblings and offspring of those whose only claim to epilepsy was a convulsion or two at the time of a childhood fever, for over 20 percent of these latter, it is said, go on later to experience other kinds of seizures.

Now if all epilepsy were grand mal in type, one might be inclined to shrug the matter off. Such an unmistakable convulsion prompts its own immediate diagnosis and therefore the immediate institution of treatment.

But what of seizures that come in more subtle displays? Say the little seizure, petit mal? How easy for an unalerted parent to pass it off as daydreaming only —or as inattentiveness, or bids for attention—until irretrievable ground has been lost in school, in the step-by-step adjustments that growing up requires, even in self-image.

And how easy it is to call seizures of the psychomotor type by any other name—wanton acts of violence, hysteria, insanity—and, by treating the situation according to that mislabel, to deny the victim the more appropriate treatment he might have gotten had he or someone in his family been forewarned.

And then there are the seizures emanating from those reaches of the nervous system that call the rhythm of one's organs. Those parts of the nervous sytsem that govern the nitty-grit of organ functions in behalf of the thinking brain that the state of consciousness might be reserved for loftier things. Should sweating, or flushing, or tearing of the eyes, or abdominal pain and vomiting occur *with* frank convulsions, their nature is rarely in doubt. But should they by chance occur in isolation, who would necessarily recognize their epileptic nature—given the extreme abundance of such complaints on nonepileptic grounds—no matter how severe they be, how frequent their attacks, or how disconcerting to the victim? Recognition might be harder still if attacks should mimic, as they often do, such things as simple acute anxiety, off-and-on neuroses or even acute appendicitis.

Epilepsy which is purely of this form most certainly exists. That woman in the Sussex garden was a case in point, her seizure being a harmless enough disturbance in the rhythm of her heart and circulation. And that fevered five-year-old in Sydney was another. In his case, the seizure was the fever itself.

For the close blood relative of the epileptic, then, any troublesome symptom which begins and ends abruptly, which keeps recurring, and which cannot be explained on other more obvious grounds should be regarded with suspicion. Chances are the problem will turn out to be not epilepsy at all. But if it *is,* that healthy suspicion could well be the shortest path by far to appropriate treatment and relief.

Now no discussion of epilepsy would be complete without a reference to that controversial villain, migraine headache.

Is it—or is it not—epileptic?

There are those who claim that epilepsy and migraine are totally unrelated. And there are those— some notable authorities among them—who believe that migraine is a seizure originating from those portions of the nervous system that have to do with organ function.

Correspondingly, there are studies that show an undue frequency of migraine among the relatives of epileptics and of epilepsy among the relatives of those who suffer migraine. And there are studies, on the other hand, which show no such correlation.

There seems to be no question, however, that migraine, regardless of its nature, is a lot more prevalent than epilepsy per se, that its heritability is a good deal more pronounced, and that the major risk it imposes on the next of kin is for more of the very same thing: migraine itself.

All in all, then, there is much about epilepsy that we have yet to learn.

And the pursuit of that knowledge is more or less everyone's concern. For the privilege of being epilepsy-free accrues only to individuals, never to families. In every family, sooner or later—like varicose veins, like schizophrenia, like *any* common disorder—epilepsy appears.

As it was present in the ancestry of all human beings alive today, so it is destined to appear in the descendency of us all. Assuming only two or three children per family, in fact, the chance of seizures among that clan consisting only of one's children, grandchildren, and great grandchildren is, on an average, over 25 percent. And that figure is low, for not all seizures are recognized as such. If all were recognized, the figure would likely be well over 50 percent.

It is a figure sufficiently high, in other words, to make three generations from now—say, seventy-five years hence—a tempting deadline for the final achievement of what we have yet to learn in the way of epilepsy's cause and control and prevention.

Still—is that not perhaps an overly ambitious goal? Consider how much we have yet to learn about the brain itself and the fantastic challenges that its complexity imposes.

Is the brain decipherable at all?

Are there certain features of life, perhaps even of illness itself, beyond human ken and control?

Put the question to Hippocrates.

Let one ask the master physician, if he dare—

"Is it not likely that the human brain is too complex to comprehend?"

"Too complex for comprehension?" Can one not almost see the impatience twinkling now in those sharp old eyes. "Well, and that is an old familiar tune I seem to have heard before. But this time what an alibi it is that it traps itself. If the human brain be truly that complex—in the name of Zeus—all the better then to understand it with!"

IX

The Rh Factor

As an animal behaves, so, often, does a cell. Many of the instincts that govern the one, govern also the other. And the rejection of that which is *different* is a classical example.

Now *what* is different must be learned, of course. But the subject is easily mastered. "Different" is simply that with which an individual, through lack of exposure early in life, has not become familiar.

Thus it happens that a baby duck, tended from its first few hours of life by a loving mother cat, grows up to be itself a cat, in its own eyes at least, with naught but a hiss, should their paths later happen to cross, for its own biologic mother. Even sex may not be sufficient to dissuade it. Come mating season, it will likely waste its energies mooning after another cat.

The fact of it is, then, that ducks regard them-

selves as ducks, and cats as cats, and man as man because their earliest exposures happened to be, respectively, to creatures of that kind.

In the same way, precisely, does a cell, early in
the embryonic life of its host, come to learn what is
and is not alien. Beyond that point in time any other
cell or cellular substance to which that embryo host
has not yet been exposed is declared forever foreign.
Different. A potential enemy, subject, if ever encountered, to the full fury of its host's cellular
defenses.

The compulsion both of animal and cell to reject
all things that are unfamiliar has without a doubt
been a boon to the survival of every complex species.
For, overall, such action tends to be protective.

It is this compulsion, after all, that keeps a bird
from too glibly consorting with cats, or insects from
consorting with birds. Or man, at one time perhaps,
from accepting with too much abandon the company
of tigers.

Undoubtedly, such rejection has also had a pur-
gative effect on the collective genes of various animal
species. Ignorant though a mother dog may be of
what prompts her, for example, to destroy her own
defective pups, her act assures that whatever genes
may have been at fault are removed from species
circulation.

No less protective is the rejecting behavior of
the cells themselves. Were they not to be nettled by
chance encounters with certain bacteria, say, or
viruses, who knows in what primeval graveyard most
of the animal kingdom might be lying today? One's

recovery from smallpox or measles, for example, is dependent on his cells' ability to recognize the invading virus as alien and through the production of antibodies—chemical soldiers, as it were, custom-made for the virus in question—to destroy it.

Now it stands to reason that such an instinct, to be fully effective, must be sensitive enough that it rarely allows for exceptions.

And that sensitive it obviously is.

But highly sensitive devices—those that nature designs in moments of pragmatic inspiration, at least —command big prices.

If aliens are invariably to be recognized as such, not even those that are innocent can be afforded the benefit of a doubt—including those that only *seem* to lack familiarity, because of some angular perspective, say, or a certain lighting, or as a result perhaps of some distortion in the eyes of the beholder.

So it is also that a highly sensitive and serviceable device, to assure that none of the guilty will go undamned, backfires now and then—at both levels, animal and cell.

The human being is a notable example. To that category of "alien, potentially hostile environment" he assigns not only bears and snakes and various versions of Martians but certain innocents as well—certain of his own kind—whose unfamiliar customs, colors of skin, values, or faiths play red herring to his instinct to reject.

It is sensitivity at the price of specificity, then. A kind of over-kill.

If race discrimination, for example, seems to be

unreasoning, that is simply because it *has* no basis in reason. Its basis is instinct, misapplied. Since the human being is intelligent enough to recognize an instinct for what it is, however, he is also capable of redirecting it to that purpose for which it is more properly intended. If man still practices race discrimination then, even if only in his heart, it is not for lack of intelligence; it is for failure to use it.

Unfortunately, the cell has no such intellectual powers. And it, like man, is all too often guilty of instinct-misguided behavior.

The epitome of such indiscretions are those reactions—the so-called auto-immune diseases, like rheumatoid arthritis and a host of others—in which an individual inadvertently takes to custom-making antibodies against himself. That is, against one or another of his own highly specialized tissues.

Still, there is no denying that that calamitous disease of the unborn child—induced by what is commonly called the *Rh factor*—is an even more poignant example of the fallability of instinct. For in effect it represents a mother, against her will, turned against her child.

Or more specifically, it represents a mother taken to making antibodies against the red cells in her child's blood. Against that substance, the Rh factor, in the child's cells which her own red cells, lacking the substance themselves, have haplessly labeled "alien." And that, in spite of the fact that the presence of the Rh substance is more characteristic of the human species than is its absence, for only a minority of most populations—usually less than 17 percent—are found to lack it. To be Rh *negative,* that is. And in certain groups, Orientals in particular, that figure plummets to something close to zero.

For the infant under attack, the result can be anything from death in the womb to a mild, short-lived anemia that does not develop until after birth. Without treatment, severely affected infants born alive usually die in a matter of hours or days and those who survive bear such unmistakable battle scars as deafness, retardation, and spastic or paralyzed muscles—the results of a toxic accumulation in the infant's brain of the "pigment spill," so to speak, from too many red cells shattered to bits by those maternal missiles launched from the mother's circulation.

Now an Rh negative infant, of course, cannot induce a mother to such antibody-making, since it, too, lacks the alien substance. Nor, for the same reason, can such an infant be affected by antibodies the mother may already have made as a result of a previous Rh *positive* child.

It is a peculiarity of this desease, moreover, that the *first* Rh positive infant of an Rh negative mother is also never affected, or only rarely so. Ordinarily, during pregnancy, there is not sufficient contact between the mother's and the unborn infant's blood to arouse her cellular defenses. It is rather during delivery, when the efforts of the womb to empty itself often force appreciable amounts of an infant's blood into the mother's circulation, that the mother's cellular intelligence—retrospectively—classifies the child as alien.

Belatedly, after her infant has escaped the womb, her cellular defenses set about the business of antibody-making, with no harm done were it not for the fact that unused Rh antibodies, unfortunately, are never discarded as obsolete. They are kept, in waiting, for the duration of a mother's life, ready for action with every Rh positive child she subsequently carries. And while the placenta—that tissue barrier, sometimes called the "after-birth," that lies between an unborn infant and its mother—is rather effective in preventing the mingling of their bloods, it is notoriously facile at giving Rh antibodies carte blanche admission to an infant's circulation.

Rh disease—the devastation itself that is wrought in the infant—is genetically based only in the sense that one's Rh status, positive or negative, is a strictly inherited matter.

And it is an altogether dominant gene that determines the presence of the Rh factor, and hence the positive Rh status. Should the carrier of such a gene, by virtue of inheritance from his other parent, carry the gene for Rh negativity as well, he will be positive in spite of all, and all his red cells will contain the Rh factor. Unlike the carrier of naught but positive genes, however, he offers his offspring a fifty-fifty chance of inheriting either one. Should such an offspring, opting for the negative gene, receive a similar contribution from his other parent, he will of course turn out to be an Rh negative infant, as *all* the children must be who are born to Rh negative couples.

For the Rh negative wife of an Rh positive husband, then, the chance at any pregnancy of an Rh negative child—with all that that implies in the way of peaceful coexistence—is either 50 percent or nil. It all depends on whether or not her husband hosts an Rh negative gene.

Rh testing is routinely done in so many situations now that it is not at all uncommon for one to know his Rh status even though his interest in the finding is purely academic. Indeed, the test is simple enough that the students of any biology class could undertake it as an easy laboratory exercise.

It is even possible, in more expert hands, to determine whether an Rh positive person has only positive genes or a positive-negative mix. To decide, that is, which of those two alternative chances, 50 percent or nil, is actually the case.

Even the more hazardous of these situations, however—that combination of an Rh negative wife and a husband with only Rh positive genes—does not necessarily spell trouble. Given the frequency of such matings—14 percent of couples—the wonder may be that the incidence of affected infants is so low, less than one out of every two hundred births.

Obviously then, mere incompatibility in a couple's Rh status is not sufficient to produce the disease.

In the first place, unless enough of an infant's red cells stray across the placenta to trespass on maternal grounds, the mother's cellular defenses will not be triggered into antibody production. And though such "leakage" is common, the number of trespassers is often too slight to be noticed.

In the second place, some women seem to have a natural gift for making antibodies whose function, oddly enough, is to inhibit antibody-making. How helpful this trait is in preventing Rh disease has yet to

be confirmed but it could explain why certain Rh negative women seem to be able to bear any number of Rh
positive infants without untoward effect. It might also
explain why certain Rh negative women do not make
antibodies in spite of significant leakage.

And then there is that twist of circumstance in
which a bad situation, by getting worse, gets better. This
kind of situation occurs in the Rh negative woman who
is incompatible with her Rh positive husband on yet
another score, being of blood type "O" while his blood
type is "A."

Now the individual of blood type O comes endowed at birth—no prior contact needed—with antibodies against that substance "A" that the red blood
cells of type A persons all contain. In the serum of the
type O individual, there are missiles already made and
waiting, then, for any chance encounter with alien
blood, whether from a mismatched transfusion bottle
or from a "mismatched" infant's circulation.

And it is that, exactly, that can save the would-be
affected infant from the blight of Rh disease. For if,
like its father, the infant is of blood type A, no sooner
do its red cells stray across the placenta onto maternal
grounds than they are pounced upon by her antibodies-
against-the-substance "A" and destroyed beyond all recognition. Destroyed before the mother's cellular defenses have had an opportunity to detect any equally
alien Rh substance they might have contained.

It is true, of course, that the infant suffers red cell
loss in either case. But the damage done by the incompatibility between blood types O and A is ordinarily
mild, if discernable at all.

Among Rh negative women who have had at least one Rh positive child, then, the risk to future children is at least partly presaged by what has gone on before.

If such a mother has yet to have an affected infant, the hazard at each new pregnancy is only 5 to 10 percent. Once she has suffered that misfortune, though, recurrence is the rule, and the risk to each future positive child may approach 100 percent. Moreover, since Rh antibodies last in the mother for life, it helps not one iota to try to wait them out.

It is ironic in a way, now that the means exist for preventing the formation of antibodies to begin with, that those herculean efforts needed to save the already blighted child should still be so often required.

For thousands of women around the world, however, that ingenious technique came a pregnancy too late. For their infants, of course, such herculean efforts —massive transfusions which completely replace a newborn's blood with blood that is antibody-free, or transfusions even prior to birth through the wall of the mother's abdomen and womb—can make the difference between life and death. Or make the difference between a grossly disabled and a relatively normal child.

But, by comparison, that means of preventing trouble to begin with is so simple that it borders on the elegant.

At the birth of a positive infant, the Rh negative mother is merely given an injection of the very thing one does not want her to have: antibodies against the Rh factor.

However contradictory that procedure may seem, it is based on sheer and simple logic. Since most of the leakage of an infant's red cells into a mother's circulation occur at the time of birth, Rh antibodies deliberately injected at this time fall upon such alien cells and, like those antibodies-against-the-substance-A, destroy them literally hours before they have a chance to arouse the suspicion of a mother's antibody-making defense.

Now it is a twist with a twist perhaps that the antibodies injected, being not of the mother's own making, being "alien" in a sense, are shortly banished from her blood. And there is nary a trace of one left to pose any threat by the time she is pregnant again.

With each succeeding birth of an Rh positive infant, even prematures and stillbirths, the risk recurs, of course, and treatment must therefore be repeated. Under this regimen, however, each and every Rh positive infant that a negative mother bears is just as secure as if he were her first.

On occasion, if there is evidence that significant leakage has occurred, this technique is used even while a mother is pregnant. For while the dosage of the injection is sufficient to prevent her from making antibodies of her own, it is apparently too low to have any effect on the infant.

Since the technique is effective only where self-made antibodies do not already exist, it goes without saying, of course, that the Rh negative female—at *any* age, pregnant or not—should never, in the event of transfusion, be given Rh positive blood. Under such circumstances, even her *first* Rh positive infant may have no protection at all.

The same rationale underlies that caution that a

woman never be given her husband's blood. Even to
the Rh positive woman this caution applies, for her
husband's blood may well contain some variant factor,
not routinely tested for, that could provoke an antibody
response. In such a case, any of her subsequent infants
who inherited that variant from its father would be
subject to assault.

Now such precautions, by and large, including the
use of preventive antibody treatment, are already a part
of professional routine.

There are certain initiatives, however, that can be
taken only by the Rh negative woman herself.

It is she, for example, who in seeking prenatal care
determines how early in her pregnancy surveillance
shall begin. And the sooner that surveillance is begun,
of course, the sooner any untoward event, however
unusual, can be detected and corrected.

The second initiative has to do with abortions, or
rather their prevention. For the induced abortion—far
more than natural miscarriage—is liable to cause mass
leakage of an embryo's cells into a mother's circulation.
Whether or not such leakage is as provocative of
maternal antibody production as that occurring during
birth is not yet clear. But so long as the potential exists,
one must presume the hazard is there.

Antibody injection, of course, will effectively prevent that misfortune, and indeed is recommended for
all Rh negative women undergoing abortion. All the
same, it is one more thing to have to consider, and one
more thing to have to pay for, at a time when both the
mother and her financial situation are often already
under strain.

If pregnancy prevention is preferable to abortion for *any* woman, it is even more so, then, for the Rh negative girl. Moreover, the abundance of contraceptive choices available today give her no dearth of opportunity to exercise that discretion.

All in all, then, it is only a matter of time before Rh disease is literally made to disappear.

Already the incidence has begun to drop. And that decline will become increasingly precipitous as more and more antibody-hosting women, passing out of child-bearing age, are replaced with those who, by virtue of treatment, are still antibody-free.

As a matter of fact, eradication of Rh disease could well be achieved within the span of a single generation. Could be made to end abruptly—after leaving a trail who knows how many eons long—in one short, terse finale. With one last incisive mention in the human diary—asterisked, of course, lest future generations fail to see that crucial warning at the bottom of the page.

The cautionary footnote reminding one and all that if vigilance is not maintained, without a doubt history will repeat.

For, as a result of treating Rh disease, Rh negative genes will be even more abundant in the future than they are right now. And as long as the instinct to reject safeguards the destiny of animals and cells, so must their individual members be prone to such perceptual errors as turn them, viciously if inadvertently, against others of their kind.

X

Birth Defects

THAT 97 PERCENT of infants are born apparently normal is testimony not to the perfection of the human stock but rather to nature's diligence in weeding the garden of human conceptions. By the highest estimates, one out of five such conceptions is so grossly blighted that that venerable abortionist herself strikes it from the running, often so quickly that the would-be mother may not be aware she was pregnant.

Thus, with relentless surveillance, does nature conceal from man his true potential for misdesign.

By the time of birth, defective infants constitute only 3 percent of the total of live births. A good share of those defects, moreover, are apparently nowhere serious enough at that, in nature's eyes at least, to merit disqualification.

A survey of living infants only, then, admittedly gives a somewhat diluted version of the maladies that lurk along the road between conception and that ultimate expatriation known as birth.

But the evidence gleaned from stillbirths, 15 percent of which are visibly defective—and from miscarried embryos as well—does tend to support what one must infer from that residual 3 percent of live births that are defective: of the myriad afflictions of the yet-to-be-born, so-called *malformations*—architectural defects, as it were—top the list.

Given the intricacy of parts that go into the making of a child, given the fastidious timetable by which the growth of each part must be geared to the growth of the rest, it is not surprising perhaps that malformations are so common.

That malformations as a group have no simple, single cause, is equally unsurprising.

Infections like German measles, for example, have no respect for the membrane barrier that separates an unborn infant from its mother. And infection is a notorious saboteur of the process of orderly growth, as are certain drugs that a mother might happen to take.

The placenta, moreover—that so-called "afterbirth" through which the unborn infant negotiates to meet the gamut of his needs—is not immune to disorders of its own. Nor is it necessarily above anchoring onto some inauspicious portion of the womb.

Even a child's genes can act to invite an architectural disaster. For though the truly common malformations—say those that occur in one or more of every thousand births—are rarely worded as defects *per se* in the blueprint specifications of a child's heredity, there is little doubt that certain genes do not observe the safety standards of the biologic building code.

There is also no doubt, however, that the chance of recurrence of the same malformation in subsequent children is relatively low. Much lower, as a matter of fact, than people sometimes think, particularly those who happen to be the parents of a malformed child and, more particularly, if that child happens to be their first and as yet only offspring. For it is only natural that one be blinded to what *might* have happened by what actually *did*.

Now, oddly enough, it is the very abundance of genes required to produce such malformations that tends to keep the risks from getting out of hand.

No job as complex as synchronizing organ growth, of course, could be carried out by anything less than a literal orchestra of genes. Performed in unison, the separate renditions of such genes act to establish the threshold, so to speak, which environmental insults must exceed to interfere with orderly organ growth. Thresholds that are low enough to be exceeded by the everyday insults of an ordinary environment seem to depend on such a special genetic combination—like a flush in poker—that the odds are against such thresholds occurring even if the parents, between them, carry all the necessary genes. This state of affairs explains why malformations—no less than musical genius—are so much harder to come by than traits whose presence depends on a choice between one gene or the other of a single parental pair.

In *harelip,* for example—regardless of whether or not the palate, or the roof of the mouth, is also cleft—the risk of recurrence in a subsequent child is roughly 5 percent, and in the offspring of an affected parent only 2 or 3 three percent. The risk, then, is a good deal less than the 25 or 50 percent risk so typical of traits that are due to a single gene or a pair.

In *cleft palate* alone, the risk of a second affected infant is 1 to 2 percent, and 7 percent for the offspring of a parent who was himself affected.

In the case of *club foot,* the risk of recurrence in a subsequent child is similarly low—somewhere in the neighborhood of 3 percent.

Even that most serious of all common malformations, "open spine" or *spina bifida*—that defect in which the backbone, failing to close, allows the spinal cord to herniate externally—carries with it a risk to subsequent children of 5 percent. That figure applies, however, only to infants who are born alive. A certain percentage of affected live births, moreover, will not have spina bifida but *anencephaly* instead—a deficiency of skull and brain formation incompatible with life.

In *pyloric stenosis*—stomach muscle overgrowth which, if productive of obstruction, only surgery can undo—the threshold effect is more dramatically apparent because of the fact that the defect is five times more common in boys than in girls. Such a difference would be only natural of course if girls, to be affected, required a greater number of "low threshold" genes. In this case the parents of affected daughters could be expected to harbor more of such genes than the parents, on an average, of only affected sons. In which case, in turn, the risk of recurrence should be greater among the future offspring of the former.

And that is precisely what one sees. In the families

of affected daughters the average risk per offspring is 9 percent—over twice the 4 percent recurrence rate seen in the families of only affected sons. Moreover, the highest risk of all should accrue specifically to the brothers of affected girls, which it does indeed. Their chance of pyloric stenosis, 15 percent, tops all the rest.

In malformations of the *heart*—granted the high proportion of cases accounted for by environment alone —the overall risk of recurrence in subsequent children, though severalfold the average, is still only 2 percent.

Even a *combination* of defects does not necessarily imply a high genetic risk. For subsequent siblings of multiply-malformed infants the chance of a repeat is less than 3 percent.

Low though such risks may be, however—at least as risks in heredity often go—the truth of it is that beyond controlling known environmental offenders, there is relatively little that can yet be done to make such risks any lower.

Only rarely, or only under most exceptional conditions, can the presence of malformation be detected in an unborn child. Nor would we—if through some gift of periscopic vision we could observe a malformation in the making—have the fuzziest notion of how to circumvent it. There is some compensation, however, in the fact that most of the common malformations are often so readily apparent at or shortly after birth that appropriate treatment tends to suffer little delay.

There are certain crucial exceptions.

Among the truly common malformations there are two, hip dislocation and defects of the urinary system, which, like those above, can be disastrous if untreated. But, *un*like the rest, they are highly likely to escape one's notice until irremediable damage has been done.

DISLOCATION OF THE HIP

Dislocation of the hip is a misnomer, really. The actual defect is merely an over-laxness of the joint or a somewhat shallow socket, and dislocation is rather the end result. Along with its disabling deformation of the joint, dislocation is the very object of prevention.

This defect is, moreover, notably selective—preferring girls to boys, one hip to two, left side to right. Likewise it has a preference for wintertime debuts. And its disaffinity for Negroes and Chinese is as unabashed as is its penchant for Lapps and Navajos.

Still, neither sex nor race nor weather makes one totally immune. And if dislocation seems ethnically inclined, it is due not so much to ethno-oriented genes as it is to the fact that man is a creature of habit.

The genes after all do nothing more than predispose a child to dislocation by causing joint laxity or shallowness of socket.

Take the geneticists' favorite subject, a pair of identical twins. Where one twin has hip dislocation, in only 40 percent of such pairs does the other one, too. Since identical twins have identical genes, to the environment alone must go full credit for the other 60 percent.

Neither is there any doubt, however, that full credit for the predisposition must go to the genes. For an X ray of the normal twin will invariably reveal the predisposing defect, as will an X ray of the normal hip of a child whose dislocation is one-sided.

Among the siblings of a child with dislocation, it is therefore not surprising that 5 percent suffer similar dislocation, as do 5 percent of the offspring of a dislocated parent, and 10 to 15 percent of infants with *both* a sibling and parent affected.

Now frank dislocation tends to develop sometime after birth. Silently, without symptoms. Often unsuspected until a child, learning to walk, is observed to waddle like a duck.

And by then it is too late.

For if a child with dislocation is not treated by six months of age, even the best of surgery, it is said, however it improves his plight, cannot give him back a normal joint. And there is no guarantee that what improvement is achieved can be indefinitely maintained. Years later, troublesome symptoms may reappear, and throughout his life he will be subject to arthritis of the hip.

Contrast that plight with the result of treatment which prevents the dislocation to begin with. Such treatment is made totally feasible today by virtue of the fact that the predisposition itself can now be readily detected. In the hands of someone practiced in the technique the test takes less than a minute. And if done within twenty-four hours after birth, it rarely if ever misses.

Sometimes called the "click" test, it consists of a skillful maneuvering of a newborn's hips to elicit that tell-tale sound which marks him dislocation-prone.

So reliable is the test, it is said, that were it done

on every newborn as a matter of routine—as it is now, by strict requirement, in Sweden—the problem of permanent disability due to actual dislocation would largely disappear. For a positive test results routinely in treatment.

Granted, not all such infants would necessarily have suffered dislocation. But there is no way of telling beforehand which infants those will be. And waiting to see if dislocation develops can only end up penalizing those who are not that lucky.

Besides, that preventive treatment is so simple. With a pillow or like contrivance the thickness of a dozen diapers, the infant's legs are kept apart with hips in a slightly flexed position. That position, plus gentle stretching of the hips at every diaper change until the infant is one-year-old, practically assure a normal joint.

In effect the practice is nothing more than what many a parent does in deference not to the fear of dislocation but to the force of cultural habit.

Recall for a moment the Chinese mother's age-old custom of carrying her infant on her back. Visualize that typical piggy-back perch—infant nestled in its sling, hips flexed, legs akimbo, one leg off to either side —and guess the truth behind that disaffinity that dislocation of the hip displays for certain populations.

Then contrast that with another common custom —the swaddling of an infant, mummy-style, legs straight and rigidly together—and guess the truth also behind dislocation's favoritism for Navajos and Lapps.

Or consider for a moment how in that same protective fashion *any* mother *any*where might tend to swaddle her infant during the colder months of the year. And hypothesize—as even the professionals must, not really knowing—that dislocation's predilection for wintertime debuts is due perhaps to something just that simple.

Let he who puts too much stock, then, in any one of the elements—the genes, environment, or culture—be minded of that fallacy by dislocation's example.

For it illustrates so nicely the often forgotten truth that what man is and does depends on no one element alone. And no more on the lot of them together than on what, in their obligate interdependence, they inevitably do unto each other.

MALFORMATIONS OF THE URINARY SYSTEM

There is a generous leeway for error in the human design.

And fortunately so. Else one out of every ten of us would succumb rather sooner than we should from urinary malformations alone. From such defects as strictures, mispositions, and duplication or absence of indispensable parts anywhere along the tract from kidneys through urethra.

The frequency with which such malformations turn up unexpectedly in the autopsies of older people who died of altogether unrelated causes, however, is testimony to the body's ability to adapt to even major deviations from the normal design.

Unfortunately, not *all* malformations lend themselves to such peaceful negotiation. Those in particular that are given in any way to obstructing the flow of urine are particularly mal-inclined. For impedence anywhere along the tract is an invitation to infection. And infection, or even the backward pressure generated by the obstruction itself as a matter of simple hydraulics, can lead to progressive kidney damage.

Certain malformations—strictures, for example, and contractures of the bladder neck—are notorious producers of obstruction. But any misplacement or duplication of parts that throws a kink into the urinary plumbing can have the same effect.

If the mechanics of urinary defects are fairly well understood, however, their heritability most certainly is not. True, certain types of defect do seem more subject to genetic influence than do others. But systematic studies of inheritance are so few and far between that any attempt to individualize by malformation type is more revealing of our ignorance than productive of meaningful risks.

As yet, one can say with confidence only that the contributions of the genes are frequent enough, or forceful enough, to impart to the group as a whole a definite family bent. The tendency of urinary defects to aggregate in certain families is enough to have prompted a plea from the urologic specialists themselves for an all-out study of hereditary factors.

In lieu of anything specific to go on, then, one must simply assume that all of the offspring and siblings of anyone with any kind of urinary malformation are at some increased risk of urinary problems. And if that assumption turns out eventually to be too generous, it will at least have had the virtue of erring on the safer side. For the penalty of missing a case may be permanent kidney damage with all its attendant problems, including possibly death.

It is of no small consequence, therefore, that harmful urinary malformations usually give fair warning well in advance of kidney damage.

The problem of early detection is not a dearth of signs. It is the abandon, rather, with which such signs often mimic more or less exactly those of any of a number of other less harmful situations.

By far and away the most common warning signal is urinary infection—most often showing up as painful urination, even fever, and on occasion, persistent back or abdominal pain. Chronic infection, particularly—or acute infections which tend to recur after cessation of antibacterial drugs—are suggestive of malformation. Among school-age children with chronic infection, for example, 60 percent have been found to have underlying obstruction due to developmental defects in the urinary tract.

Problems in voiding, such as chronic bed wetting, infrequent or difficult urination, may also signal underlying obstruction. Even a failure to thrive or gain weight, especially in infants may be an indication.

The point to be made is this. In the high risk child or young adult any such signs, however innocent they may seem, deserve a high degree of suspicion.

If malformation is present, and detection not delayed past the point of irreversible danger, the outlook is generally so favorable that it more than justifies that extra-thing-to-have-to-think-about that a little vigilance entails. For between surgery and the antibacterial drugs, the vast majority of obstructive malformation can be either cured completely or rectified to the point where normal kidney function can be indefinitely maintained.

The at-risk child then is truly no cause for alarm. And that modicum of watchful awareness he requires, more often than not, will turn up nothing at all. If out of every ten such parents who maintain that watch, however, nine need not have bothered, who would deny it will have been a vigilance worth keeping?

With notable success, then, man does manage now and then to redesign his built-in imperfections. And, with time, he seems bound to undertake the redesign of an increasing number of such imperfections.

Within certain limits, it is true. No one, willingly, would retrieve from the graveyard of human conceptions that one out of five human embryos so grossly blighted that it died in the process of beginning. At least no one who treasures the right of a child to take some measure of enjoyment in his own existence.

But neither can man resist the temptation to make improvements in such of his malformations as nature leaves to his discretion. For he knows—if not consciously, instinctively at least—that it is always *imperfection* which poses the challenge.

Once universally achieved, even the normal human design must arbitrarily become a subject for critical contemplation. For the substance of so-called perfection is but a mirage. An illusion.

Perfection *has* no substance.

It is rather a *direction*. And imperfection is but the fuel to pursue it.

"When a woman gives birth to an infant that has

no fingers," the Babylonians wrote, "the town will have no births."

It is inscribed so on tablets of stone.

"When a woman gives birth to an infant that has no right nostril, the people of the world will be injured."

"When a woman gives birth to an infant that is perfect in the eyes of the world"—or so the inscriptions might have read and been closer to the truth—"then it will signify not that the world will come to a stop but that it has stopped already."

Perfection, after all, is the carrot on the stick. And the little boy was right.

"Why is it, do you think," his grandfather teased, "that Mr. Donkey never eats the carrot?"

"Because," said the little boy—being far too young to let the obvious decoy him—"he wouldn't, if he ate it, have anywhere to go."

XI

Mental Retardation

THE ROAD TO genetic distinction—to specieshood, as it were—is always a one-way street.

Evolution may take a species down a path it would rather not have traveled. May lure it over high cliffs deep into the canyons of extinction. Entice it into stagnant waters, or push it out to shoot the rapids of accelerated change.

But never, so far as we know, does evolution allow a species to retrace its steps, either to the shelter of any of its own past forms or to the entrance, via a fork in the road behind, to a path since traveled by any other species.

The rule is binding on individuals as well, and on all such complex traits—like mentality and behavior—that serve as species trademarks.

The point is so obvious it would hardly merit mention were it not for the fact it is so often overlooked.

How common, for example, is that glib assumption that feeble-mindedness is but a slipping down the ladder of species mentalities to another, lower rung.

Nothing could be further from the truth.

The mentality of the retarded child, for all his retardation, is uniquely human. His is not an inferior brain. It is a *damaged* brain, a damaged *human* brain. And there is no equivalence for that anywhere else on the ladder.

Now that is not to deny his problem. In truth, he is often far worse off than any creature on the rungs below. The brain of the latter—whatever its lowly blend of intellectual skills—is fully intact, equipped by the millennial efforts of its evolution to cope with its environment.

Such an environment the retarded child, in truth, could no more cope with than his own.

He is radically different, too, the damaged child, from those whose low mentality is but the tail end of nature's parceling out, within a population, of the normal variations of any complex trait. Such tail-enders, after all, are retarded only in a relative sense. Retarded only with respect to the proportion of those whose mentality is greater, or to the social complexities with which they must cope, or to the levels of skill and competence that society demands.

As such, of course, they are a normal part of the general scheme. And they will always be with us. Victims of nature's inequity perhaps, and perhaps necessarily so. For a population all of like intelligence would sooner or later perish, unless most of its individuals were willing to work enough below their potential to satisfy the diversity of tasks a healthy society still seems to require.

The damaged child, on the other hand, is an accident of nature. He represents not a frustration but an outright alteration of potential. Not only are the really severe impairments of intelligence confined to his ranks but other of his functions, beyond those measured by intelligence tests, are usually also impaired.

He is, in effect, a displaced person. Having been programmed by his evolution only for that upper rung, to exist only in a cultural milieu, he has somehow been derailed along his individual course and ended up instead in a kind of human no-man's land.

A most elusive place.

Ask any parent of a retarded child.

A somewhere place, within sight and sound and touch and still beyond reach. As if just outside the window, a parent will say. On the other side of a pane through whose immutable glass a child is forever only looking in. Though in truth the loneliness of it is the loneliness of those inside, born of pent-up thoughts, of feelings barred communication, of sentiments that must —and cannot—be conveyed.

For all of that it is a most familiar place. One to which fumbling nature exiles one out of every hundred infants born. Leaving, as a consequence, one out of every hundred parents to the over and over torment of self-inflicted questions. Including, sooner or later, the only question with any constructive intent: Will it— with what kinds of odds might it—happen again?

It is a torment more often than not unfounded, for the majority of mentally damaged children are simply

the victims of bad environmental luck—infection during pregnancy or infancy, severe birth trauma and the
like. In any such case the risk of recurrence is, therefore, little if any increased.

Even for the group as a whole—an estimated 10
percent of which are due to highly inherited defects
routinely given to playing havoc with an infant's brain
—the risk of recurrence in a subsequent child is only
3 percent.

Within that 10 percent, to be sure, the risks are
consequential, tending to run as high as 25 percent or
even higher, depending on the causative disorder.

Disorders contributing to this category are legion,
however. And when the 10 percent is parceled up accordingly, the number one villain among them, best
known by its initials, PKU, accounts for a scant 1 percent of all retarded children.

Of the other multitudinous disorders in which retardation is routine and heritability has any role at all,
there is only one which qualifies as common.

Common enough, at least, that its victim does not
lack for familiarity even to those who pay but the
slightest attention to children. For he is one out of
every six hundred born and, by and large, no longer
concealed in institutions. Increasingly now one sees him
playing in his own front yard, or the neighborhood
park—or trundling off to school, even if in special
buses, even if to special classes, even if for schooling
in other than the 3-R skills.

Moreover he is not easy to mistake. For the stamp
of his affliction is remarkably consistent: the tranquil
countenance, the supple-jointedness that goes with lack

of muscle tone, the almond eyes resembling from a distance those of the race for which the malady was named—*mongolism.*

For its obvious vulnerability to racist misinterpretation, it is an inappropriate name.

Other labels have been tried, without success. "Down's disease," for instance, to honor the physician —or possibly to spite him—who, in naming mongolism to begin with, started all the ruckus.

"Mongolism," then, continues to prevail. Someday perhaps a better term will come along, one appealing enough to overcome the incumbency advantage that keeps "mongolism" in terminologic office.

As a rule, the mongoloid child is rather severely retarded. That he is often as alert as any other infant in the first few months of life is a cruel peculiarity of this disease, for it frequently arouses in a parent hopes that time will almost certainly dash. Over the next two years his intellectual deficit becomes increasingly apparent. On intelligence tests his ultimate IQ score is usually less than fifty. He is generally more trainable than educable, then, and only very rarely self-supporting.

And that is strange because, in every genetic sense of the word, the mongoloid child is superendowed.

To understand such a thing, however, one must first consider the innards of a cell. Specifically, the chromosomes themselves. Those literal life boats, as it were, that house the genes throughout the course of life and ferry them over the choppy channels between succeeding generations.

Normally, there are twenty-three pairs of boats in

all, each pair the pooled contribution of one's parents.

So it is for *body* cells, at least. For *sex* cells only half as many life boats is the rule, each sex cell carrying but a singleton from each and every pair. It is necessarily so. Were an ovum and a sperm each to carry the entire fleet, the fertilized egg resulting from their union would host not twenty-three chromosomal pairs but twenty-three quadruplets. And those twenty-three quadruplets would of course persist in each of the millions of cells that the fertilized egg is destined to produce in its own image.

An extravagant blunder that would be deemed theoretical only until the report, a few years back, of an actual case. The infant, born alive, was too grossly deformed to survive.

Clearly, then, genetic superaffluence does not make for a genetically super man.

Such errors largely come about as a result of the peculiar fashion in which a cell, to multiply, divides. Using the chemicals in its larder to fabricate a duplicate set of chromosomal pairs, a body cell—say a cell in the liver or muscle or skin—then separates one such set from the other sufficiently to split in half between them.

Because its product is simpler, perhaps, the cell that generates ova or sperm observes a ritual more elaborate. In effect, however, it simply cleaves its twenty-three chromosal pairs right down the middle and splits between their divided ranks becoming, as the case may be, two ova or two sperm. Each with the prerequisite number of singletons only.

With a passenger list so critical, the matter of cellular commandeering is vitally important. Should anything go wrong—should the fleet be unequally divided—any resulting ovum or sperm has dismally little to offer a mate aspiring to a healthy voyage across that choppy channel or a valid visa for the next generational shore. For most such conceptions end up in the graveyard of human beginnings. Minor miscounts included. Even those that involve but a single chromosome too many.

Exceptionally, though, nature in her weeding displays a notable laissez faire.

She is, for instance, particularly likely to be lenient toward an extra chromosome of the type making up the so-called "twenty-first" pair. Such a redundance generally results from an ovum endowed not only with its own No. 21 but inadvertently also with the one that had rightfully been its sister ovum's share. In making its own contribution of course, any normal sperm must automatically convert this dowry into a trio. A *trisomy,* so to speak. *Trisomy 21.*

In the infant itself, each and every cell of whom must repeat that chromosomal flaw, *mongolism* is the result.

Nine times out of ten, this error has neither hereditary origin nor omen.

The vast majority of cases simply reflect the exponential effect of increasing maternal age on the chance that an ovum will be so blighted.

Past thirty-five, for example, a mother is *twelve* times more likely to bear a mongoloid infant than the mother under thirty. And *seventy-five* times more so if she is over forty-five—past which maternal age, a mongoloid infant occurs at the rate of one in forty births.

Infectious hepatitis—viral infection of the liver —may have the same effect. "Epidemics" of mongoloid births, at least, have been observed to occur in the nine month wake of hepatitis outbreaks. And there is now some evidence that the blood of infected persons does indeed contain a substance that grossly disrupts the protocol of equal cell division.

Since infectious hepatitis is not a continuing phenomenon, though—and the passage of time, to the contrary, is relentlessly so—the risk of a mongoloid birth to a mother who has already had a mongoloid child, in the majority of cases, is about the same as the risk to *any* mother *of a corresponding age.*

It is only in that minority estimated as 10 percent of cases of trisomy 21 that the risk of recurrence is increased on hereditary grounds. For in this residue of cases, the affected infant signifies the culmination, a generation delayed, of an unnegotiable error in a parent's own design.

Such an infant is the tragic aftermath, in other words, of a parent's close call—in the early hours of his own existence, and in spite of a thoroughly un-blemished beginning—with a similar fate.

So it can happen.

Take a normal ovum and a normal sperm and the result, of course, is a normal fertilized egg, the primor-dial cell. Let the egg begin to divide and the result is two cells, four cells, eight and so on. All of them—pro-vided things go according to Hoyle—perfect replicas of the original fertilized egg.

Suppose, though—say at the four-cell stage—one of those cells, after duplicating its No. 21 chromosomal pair in the fashion normal to such body cells, accidentally divides them not in pairs but as a triplet and a singleton instead.

Obviously the result is going to be one "mongoloid" and one "anti-mongoloid" cell. One cell with three No. 21's and the other with only one. The ultimate result, of course, will be an individual six-eighths of whose cells are normal, one eighth of whose cells are a chromosome shy, and one eighth of whose cells are the cellular stock in trade of the typical mongoloid child.

Cellularly, with respect to the twenty-first chromosome, he will be a *mosaic,* a mixture of this and that.

How many mongoloid cells such an individual hosts, and hence how many mongoloid signs he displays, will depend, of course, on how far along in his embryonic growth the cellular error occurred. The majority of mosaics, however, are relatively normal. Often so few cells are affected that the only clues are such inconsequentia as the so-called "mongoloid crease" on the palm of the hand, or certain suggestive fingerprint patterns. Or there may be no sign at all.

How much of a risk there is to the next generation, of course, depends entirely on the extent to which the ovaries or testes are affected. And that, unfortunately, is a difficult thing to determine, because the various tissues of the body are not necessarily all equally mosaic. That the cells of the skin and the blood—on which, for technical reasons, the diagnosis must ordinarily be made—show a certain frequency of trisomic cells does not mean that the sex-cell tissues are affected to a like degree. By the same token neither does an *absence* of trisomic cells in the skin and blood mean that the ovaries, or testes, are not heavily infested.

And if they are—if by chance, for example, all the ova-producing cells of an ovary, say, just happened to be trisomic—every other ovum would host an extra 21.

Tests of the skin or blood, therefore, serve only to confirm the mosaic state. They cannot be relied upon to rule it out. Nor can they, even when confirming it, be used as a comfortable yardstick of risk.

To the mosaic parent of a mongoloid child, then, one can say only that the chance of recurrence in a subsequent child is increased. How much is anybody's guess. For any one individual it could be anywhere from only slightly over average to 50 percent.

Nor will a mosaic mother's youthfulness have any dissuading effect. For the risk that mosaicism imposes is independent of maternal age.

It is a matter of no small consequence, however, that for any infant, increasing maternal age does enhance the chance of mosaicism itself, just as it does the chance of mongolism *per se*. The danger of mongolism that the older mother engenders, then, would seem to visit not only on her child but on her child's children as well.

There is yet another situation in which mongolism behaves as an inherited trait, but it is rare. Should a No. 21 chromosome break and one of its halves, in seeking reattachment, confuse an unrelated chromosome with its own missing part, the result is a strange chromosomal graft. However, since the total *amount* of each is still unchanged, no harm to the individual results. The individual who carries such a graft, however—who is, in other words, a *translocation carrier*—may have a problem on his hands the next generation around. For each of his sperm or her ova may be as likely as not, in its own formation, to wind up with the wrong combination. If the sperm or ovum is undersupplied with chromosomal matter, it dies. If oversupplied, and fertilized, the result—being tantamount to trisomy—is a mongoloid child.

Not all mongolism of the translocation type, however, is the result of a carrier parent. Perfectly normal parents can have a child with translocation mongolism if the original chromosomal break occurred in the parental ovum or sperm itself, or in the fertilized egg. Subsequent children born to such parents are at little or no increased risk.

Only 1 percent of all mongolism, as a matter of fact, is the result of a carrier parent. Though where a carrier parent is the cause, the risk of recurrence in subsequent children is not inconsequential. This is particularly true for carrier mothers, each of whom runs a 10 percent chance of a mongoloid infant at every living birth. The figure is closer to 2 percent in the case of a carrier father.

The mongoloid child himself is almost never a source of hereditary concern. No mongoloid male has ever been known to reproduce, and all are presumed to be sterile. Though mongoloid girls are sometimes fertile, less than two dozen births among them have ever been reported—half of which infants, as the chromosomal constitution of their mothers would lead one to expect, were mongoloid too.

The picture of mongolism as a whole, then, is a

mosaic in itself. It is a hodge-podge of different causes, of separate chromosomal errors, of widely disparate risks.

Out of this clutter—fortunately for the parents of a mongoloid child—the situation prevailing in any individual case can be readily singled out.

Brand new techniques—far more accurate, far less cumbersome than those first developed but a decade ago—permit not only an actual count of the chromosomes within one's cells but their identification, individually, by number. It now appears that even chromosomal *pieces,* in a cell that has suffered a chromosomal break, can be properly categorized by chromosomal source.

Carried out on the mongoloid infant, of course, such studies confirm his diagnosis beyond the shadow of a doubt. With equal facility they will reveal whether any given parent is chromosomally normal, a translocation carrier, or even, more frequently than one might expect, a mosaic.

Excepting the guesswork that mosaicism involves, it is possible, then, to pinpoint more or less exactly the risk of recurrence in any given family.

Traditionally, cost and a dearth of testing facilities have limited the application of such studies to those in whom the possibility of hereditary chromosomal error seems most likely. Namely younger mothers of mongoloid children and those with more than one affected child. The majority even of these will be chromosomally normal, their affected children simply reflecting trisomic quirks of fate.

It is only a matter of time, however, before chromosomal studies will be available to any parent of any child with a chromosomal problem.

Other than nonprocreation, there is only one option currently open to the high-risk parent seeking to avoid the birth of a mongoloid child: diagnosis early enough in pregnancy to allow for its abortion. Such diagnosis requires what is known as "amniocentesis" or the tapping—usually through the wall of a mother's abdomen and womb—of a little of the fluid that keeps an embryo afloat, and into which enough of an embryo's cells have usually strayed to allow for examination.

These cells, if obtained in adequate numbers, will almost always reveal whether an embryo is mongoloid or normal.

The procedure requires a high degree of professional skill, however, and the necessary facilities are not unlimited. The tests, therefore, have been offered primarily to the truly liable group—women over forty and women who are married to, or are themselves, either mosaics or translocation carriers.

Nonprocreation, of course, as a means of avoiding a mongoloid birth, is a highly tenable option. For the issue is more than a simple matter of whether to procreate or not. *When* to have children, for the vast majority of women, is an issue far more germane.

Consider the statistics. In that scant 11 percent of each year's total births accounted for by mothers over thirty-five lie fully half the annual contribution of brand new mongoloid infants. This source would literally wither away in nine short months if mothers were routinely to complete their families by that age.

There are certain preventive steps, then, one *can*

take. In view of the rate at which the picture of mongolism has unfolded in the last dozen years, moreover, one might well expect of the future an increased number of alternatives for action.

Some simple means of prevention, perhaps, might well be developed that would be available to all.

Or even treatment, *after* the fact.

Why not?

For expectation, consciously or otherwise, inclines the actions of the present to its purpose. Is, after all, the heart of prophesy fulfilled.

A mother chimpanzee, it is recently reported, gave birth to a mongoloid infant. And one can understand how even a mother chimpanzee might now and then—in a sudden moment of maternal contemplation, in the absence of response to her gestures of affection—truly feel a little of the "loneliness inside." But without understanding, all the same. Without resentment. And, without any real awareness of the future, with only the most primitive capacity for expectation.

In the world of the chimpanzee, then, tomorrow must forever be a rerun of today.

For these are the qualities—trademarks of that uppermost rung on the ladder of all life forms—that, in wracking, tormenting and driving man on, are the forces of purposeful change. That are the substance, it follows—and the only substance that can really be depended on—of hope itself for those of his children who have yet to be born on the other side of the glass.

XII

Of Universal and Elusive Maladies

THERE OCCURS AMONG men a disease which is viciously inherited and, if left untreated, uniformly fatal.

The heart of the problem is its victim's inability to synthesize a certain substance, a so-called "lactone," without which he cannot long survive.

There is no cure. Like the diabetic whose survival is continuously predicated on an outside source of insulin, he who suffers from this affliction must all his life continue medication or suffer a slow and painful hemorrhagic death.

Why, then, has the procreative zeal for which its victims are notorious never been dampened by either the heritability or the seriousness of this disease?

Simply because that indispensable substance is nothing more than plain old *vitamin C*. The disease resulting from its deficiency, of course, being plain, old fashioned *scurvy*. And those whose biochemical inadequacy dooms them to continual medication, comprise the entire human species.

Yet, in spite of its universality, there is no question that the trait is a defect in every sense of the word. A potential for trouble which, in bygone days at least, often came to pass. For diverse burial grounds—like those of seafarers past who did not know how pharmaceutical a well-stocked galley could be—safeguard the memory of many more men than were laid to rest by storm, or cannon, or misstep on the rigging. Moreover, out of all the animal kingdom, men and monkeys and guinea pigs are the only creatures to have lost in evolutionary transit the genetic paraphernalia for homemade vitamin C. In the general scheme of plant and animal life, they represent the exception rather than the rule. And no one has yet been able to show that any compensatory gain accrued from the loss.

Still, who would argue that anxiety over the heritability of this potentially lethal affliction would be patently absurd? Genetic susceptibility to scurvy varies so little from one individual to the next that there is literally no one to whom the recommended daily dose of vitamin C does not apply.

The point to be made is more or less self-evident. No matter how deleterious a trait, concern with its inheritance is a neurotic waste of time if the risk in affected families is so little different from that in the population at large that whatever precautions one might take are universally recommended.

What is not so evident to a good many people, however, is the fact that several far more serious scourges of contemporary man are also of this ilk, in-

cluding three of the most common, and anxiety-condu-
cive, maladies of all: *cancer, coronary heart disease,*
and *emphysema.* All three of them are disorders whose
genetic origin on the one hand and lack of hereditary
import on the other, unappreciated as that sometimes
is, justify at least their brief discussion.

CANCER

There can be no doubt that susceptibility to cancer is
in part genetically determined, for cancer is a disease
of multicellular creatures whose very multicellularity
and cellular behavior are genetically controlled.

Like susceptibility to scurvy or to measles, however, susceptibility to cancer is apparently universal.

Except in the case of a few rather rare inherited
disorders which make their victims highly malignancy-
prone, cancer behaves more in the fashion of an even-
tuality of life—escaped only by those who die too soon
of other things—than in the high-handedly preferential
manner of a well behaved hereditary trait.

Even those common malignancies whose intimated
family bent has prompted thorough study—namely,
leukemia and cancer of the breast, the stomach and the
lung—have been shown to occur with only twice the
usual frequency in the next of kin. And that increased
risk holds only for the cancer in question, for there is
no apparent tendency for cancer *per se* to aggregate in
families.

The sister of a woman with cancer of the breast,
for example, has a 10 percent chance of developing
that same malignancy by the time she is eighty-five.

The risk is 6 percent, however—nearly as impressive—for the *non*related woman.

No woman, then, can afford to take lightly that widely recommended practice of periodic self-examination of the breasts for the early detection of beginning masses or lumps. If breast cancer is detected early, the outlook is very good.

Cancer of the lung is likewise found about twice as often among the relatives of victims as in the general population. And that is not necessarily due to a heavier use of tobacco, for the *non*smoking relatives of victims seem to develop cancer of the lung slightly more often than do nonsmokers at large. Among such relatives, moreover—in contrast with the rest of the population—women are affected as often as men.

Regardless, the increase in risk that being next of kin confers is utterly trifling compared to the hazard that cigarette smoking imposes. Toss in the effects of air pollution, occupational exposures to airborne irritants and the like and the risk is nearly twenty times greater—*without* a family tendency at all—than it is for the closest of relatives who manage to avoid such things. The chance for such relatives under those conditions, by the way, is merely one in three hundred.

Among the relatives of stomach cancer victims, the risk of similar affliction is only 3 percent—scarcely double its random risk to the individual at large.

Even in that nearly invariably fatal disease, leukemia, the risk to the next of kin is only $2\frac{1}{2}$ percent, compared to the 1 percent risk all the rest of us run.

As for other common cancers—of womb or prostate gland or intestine, for example—intra-family risks are not yet clear. Studies to date have simply not been that extensive.

The mere demonstration of an increased intra-family risk, of course, does not prove that genetic factors are necessarily involved. A common family environment could also be at fault—though that, to be sure, would not reduce the risk by one iota unless one knew what the environmental agent was and could manage to avoid it.

Early detection—due in no insignificant measure to a highly enlightened public—and recent therapy advances have put a sizeable dent of late in the death rate due to cancer. By the demographic carload people are still being stricken, of course. But fewer of them are dying as a result.

Even cancer's complex blend of causes, under the high-powered lens of scientific scrutiny, has recently started to take on grain. To come into focus at diverse places for the research scientists of diverse specialties who study it now, in unison, around the world.

One of those grains looks—and behaves—for all the world like a virus.

This much is known. Certain viruses do seem to have the power to drive a cell into that state of anarchy, of restless drivenness, of wild if innovative irresponsibility, that mark it cancerous—in *certain* animals— *sometimes*. Certain viruses seem to have the power to drive a *human* cell to cancer—sometimes—in a *test tube*. Certain viruses, or antibodies against them, are found almost routinely in certain humans—with certain kinds of cancer. That any virus *is* indeed instrumental in inducing any cancer in any human has yet to be proved. The evidence is only supportive of the possibility that viruses are involved. But it is strongly supportive, and, as it collects, it is increasingly so.

At times, in certain types of cancer, the grain appears to be a chemical instead. Like an irritant, certain pollutants in the air, ingestants, or certain chemicals of occupational exposure. Or sometimes not a chemical at all but rather radiation.

Antibodies, too, or the *lack* of same. Another grain. Inadequacies of the immune response—the body's front line defense, as it were, against invasion from without and deviance within. This much we know. All cancer tissue studied is deviant enough, sufficiently chemically alien, to invite such attack. Front line defenses grow feebler, and the risk of cancer greater, with increasing age. Children with inborn defects in immune response, in antibody production, that is, or in cellular defense, have a higher incidence of cancer than do their normal peers. There are other bits of evidence too, too numerous, or nomenclaturally encumbered, for recounting here. And each provokes as many questions as it answers.

Is a cell that turns malignant, for example, an everyday phenomenon in everyone, only when the body's defenses fault—for an instant look the other way—is capable of establishing itself as cancer? Who can say? But the question is valid and it has been posed.

And what of genes? Do they sufficiently affect the vulnerability of cells to malignant persuasion by viruses, by chemicals, by radiation, to explain the minor differences seen between the unrelated and the next of kin? Or account for enough variation in immune response to produce the same thing?

A storm of questions. And questions must sooner or later beget the truth. Like a storm-spawned stream, droplet answers merge to a trickle—merge to rivulets, rivulet joining rivulet to become, sooner or later, a crescendo flow of illumination.

Somewhere downstream of the present—and possibly not too far from now—man will come to understand the nature of malignant change. Will learn to control it. Prevent it. May even learn—who knows, for the thought is surely no more irresponsible than the disease itself—to harness its wayward genius that it might be made to work to his advantage.

CORONARY HEART DISEASE

For all its indispensability the heart is a most primitive device. Its function, moreover, is relatively simple, for it does nothing more than keep the blood in motion, thus assuring the body's cells of food and oxygen and a handy self-renewing place in which to dump their wastes.

Even the pump, the heart itself—via the coronary vessels—is dependent on such catering. And nowhere else in the body is a cell's imperative for that service manifested so dramatically, so tragically, and so often.

Each year coronary heart disease claims a fresh 1 percent of our population. And those who die of it account for close to a third of the nation's yearly deaths.

Like cancer, then, it has a universal ring.

To be sure, certain environmental provokers—

smoking, nutritional indiscretions, stress and strain—have played havoc with the hearts of certain "advantaged" populations. Such provokers only serve to illustrate, however, how universal the potential really is.

Age alone is an infamous hardener of arteries—and though the environment may alter the pace, even newborns carry evidence, albeit microscopic, of having lived that long. It is the destiny of living mammalian things.

The process of arterial aging, however, does display a little individual, or *family,* variation.

Among the close blood relatives of women under sixty-five with coronary disease, the frequency of like affliction was found in one large survey to be seven-fold the average, for females and males alike.

But much under seventy at least, women are less prone than men. The disease in a younger woman, then, is likely to indicate a family with an excess concentration of high risk factors. For among affected men under fifty-five, the risk to the next of kin was found to be, for males and females respectively, five- and two-fold average.

Granted the need for further studies along this line, what does such a family aggregation probably mean?

First of all it must be understood that the "heart attack" which all too often ushers in the diagnosis is, by the time of its occurrence, indisputable evidence that coronary heart disease is already well established. And that coronary heart disease itself is but the end result of even more basic defects.

If heart attack *per se* is not directly subject to inheritance, then, neither is the state of one's coronary vessels. What *is* inherited, rather, is the rate—in any given environment—at which arteries age, and the rate, therefore, at which they approach the potential for trouble.

There is, of course, that minimum rate that nature imposes on all warm-blooded creatures, which by itself contributes heavily to the incidence of coronary disease. Progressively with increasing age.

Above and beyond that universal tendency, though, there are certain genetically influenced factors which, by speeding the process up, increase the risk of heart disease at a younger than average age. The younger the victim, therefore, the more likely it is that such a factor is involved.

High blood pressure, or *hypertension,* for example, is a notorious and common abuser of vascular give, affecting 15 percent of the population—two-thirds of which, or 10 percent of all of us, are hypertensive on hereditary grounds. Routine examination, of course, is often sufficient to detect hypertension, though periodic check-ups and, on occasion special studies, may be needed to confirm the diagnosis. Treatment generally results in good to excellent control—fortunately, for severe hypertension can play havoc with the brain and the kidneys as well.

Diabetes, too, apparently even in its early silent stages, accelerates the rate of arterial aging. As do a host of inherited metabolic maladies having to do with the handling of fat, most of which are subject to a fair degree of control through the use of special drugs and a diet tailored to the individual defect.

All these factors are more than ordinarily given to recurring in the next of kin.

The presence of those factors, coupled with the fact that families share not only certain genes but often certain habits and environments as well, is almost undoubtedly why the frequency of coronary heart disease was as high as it was in the relatives surveyed above.

For the close blood kin of the "youngish" individual with coronary heart disease, the predisposing factor, then, not heart disease itself, is the relevant thing. And it is grounds in its own right—if identifiable as an inherited trait—for examination of the next of kin. Moreover, treatment of the predisposing disorder itself—whether hypertension, diabetes, or the like—automatically whittles down the threat of coronary disease as well. Leaving its recipient in much the same predicament as anyone else—constantly having to do battle with an environment equally inclined to do our coronaries in. Having to struggle against the inimical goodies with which the environment constantly seems to tempt us, like a good cigarette, or a steady gourmet's diet. Or the scintillation—however we may consciously deny it—of the breakneck pace that "modern living," as the current dodge goes, "constantly forces us into."

EMPHYSEMA

Like cancer of the lung, emphysema has recently catapulted from the relative obscurity of a now and then, if commonly lethal, affliction to front and center status as a major medical challenge.

And for much the same reason.

Of the 12 percent of American male adults who currently suffer that progressive and destructive over-distention of the lungs that results from chronic bronchial obstruction, over 90 percent are heavy smokers. The same is true of the 1 percent of American women who are likewise emphysema victims.

Not that emphysema wields no hereditary clout. In certain individuals it does indeed, in the form of an inherited deficiency of a natural body substance, *antitrypsin*. Carriers of a double dose of the defective gene, though they are rare, seem destined to emphysema with little or no provocation, while that 5 percent of the population that carry a single such gene are unduly prone.

Regardless of how predisposed such individuals may be, the vulnerability of the remaining 95 percent of us to irreversible emphysema is sufficiently high to make the ground rules for prevention universally germane.

Who, for example, shall say that those of us who escaped the mutant gene for antitrypsin deficiency are free to smoke with any degree of impunity? Or brave for long the elements of atmospheric pollution, provocative as *they* are, too—or give callous disregard to bronchial infections till they are chronically entrenched—with such genetic liberty as would make us the envy of that 5 percent? Who shall say that anyone is genetically immune when 80 to 90 percent of all emphysema victims have managed to arrive at that state with no special genic assistance?

OF ELUSIVE MALADIES

If the universality of a trait makes its heritability an illogical object of concern, so, equally, does a lack of any recourse to prevention.

Put another way, concern with the heritability of a trait, even if nonuniversal, makes good sense only to the extent that those who are at risk can use that knowledge in self-defense.

Now there are few inherited disorders, of course, for which the art of prevention leaves nothing to be desired. And, therefore, few disorders over which concern cannot be carried to an unproductive extreme.

There are some diseases, however, that still continue to elude prevention of any kind. In such a situation almost any degree of concern translates as pure and simple worry, and worry, by definition, is a gainless pursuit.

If the risk is low of course, there may be little inclination to concern. In *cerebral palsy*, for example—impairment of muscle function due to brain damage ordinarily incurred before or during birth—hereditary causes probably account for less than 5 percent of cases. Less than 2 or 3 percent may be closer to the truth. The chance, therefore, that that misfortune would strike the random family twice is likely no greater than 1 percent.

Neither may one be inclined to concern if treatment after the fact is simple and effective. *Goitre,* or *thyroid* problems in general, for example, though elusive of prevention is so easily handled, as a rule, that its frequent heritability is rarely a family concern. Not to minimize at all the fact that a positive family history, say in a case of underactive thyroid, can expedite a diagnosis and thereby hasten symptom relief.

Even *otosclerosis*—of the myriad forms of hereditary hearing loss the only one that ranks as very common—can, if sufficiently disabling, be surgically repaired. And, if other defects do not complicate the picture, surgery nearly always gives excellent results.

Not all prevention-shy disorders, of course, can be so handily disposed of.

Take *allergy*, for instance. Indefatigable jack-in-the-box, *ad exasperatum* popping up in every generation. Or so it seems to families driven by its insistence to keeping count.

Oddly enough, however, its presence in a family is an indication only of the intrafamily risk of allergy *per se*, prophesizing nothing as to severity or type.

That the allergic parent portends a risk of 25 to 50 percent for each and every offspring must be viewed, it is true, vis-a-vis the fact that the risk is 10 percent for the child with *no* allergic parents. If the latter risk seems high, however, it is not because the environment, single-handedly, has grossly padded the account. It is rather because so many of us are silently hosting allergy genes.

Nor can allergy necessarily be written off as a minor affair. Its most serious manifestation, *asthma*—however improved by treatment—can on occasion still be chronically disabling. And even hay fever can seriously hamper one's style for weeks at a time.

Still, it is a situation more or less destined to improve. Newer and better treatment techniques will con-

inue to replace the old. Will, by definition—by intervening at progressively earlier stages—become increasingly preventive.

So it will happen eventually for all such disorders,
common and rare, that from behind the boulders of our
ignorance still taunt us with the threat of their affliction.
Just as surely as preventive measures for these elusive
maladies will come, moreover, so will bigger and better preventions for those diseases already under one
degree or another of preventive fire. Like gout, like
diabetes, like schizophrenia and the rest.

Such developments, in fact, are almost unavoidable, for in a very real sense they are happening now.
Just beyond the keyhole, as it were.

Developments whose order of realization, however—as we shall see in a moment—will best serve
those who with preconceived intent go pick-and-choos-
ing *now,* ahead of time, among the inventoried items
in the shadowed warehouse of the future.

XIII

Tomorrow through the Keyhole

IT CAN BE argued that that ever mobile element which man refers to as the "present" is but an interface between the future and the past.

Even a second, by contrast, is infinitely long. For each split second can be split in turn, indefinitely so, each smaller fragment still having a beginning and an end, the latter invariably occurring—however infinitesimally so—sometime *after* the beginning.

One simply cannot slice time thin enough, in other words, to isolate the unadulterated essence of *now*.

Whatever dimension nowness has is in the mind of its perceiver. Like the after-image of the sun persisting after one has closed his eyes, the sensations of the moment recently passed combine with the vicarious sensations of the moment yet to come—the anticipation, as it were, of certainties impending—to give the present "thickness."

Now, perceptually, stretches then from that most recent point at which past events, their after-image faded, must be recalled to be experienced again to that point in the future beyond which the element of surprise is credible enough to discourage further vicarious trespass.

For most of us—however directly the past abuts the future—the latter, then, is that territory blessed or haunted, as the case may be, by the unexpected.

A territory we may preview only through whatever token keyhole our wit and past experience allow.

Sans key, it is nonetheless a keyhole through which the whole scenario of tomorrow—should one look into that half-lit sanctum now—lies piece by piece revealed. Motions, shapes, objects—here and there in crystalline detail. As far as the eye can see—ten years hence, twenty, certain features of the timescape still boldly clear at thirty—

A revelation. Enough to reel one's head. To *see,* to *know*—precisely what?

For take another look, and another and another. And see how at every glance the features of the timescape change. How on each occasion certain objects have been added or deleted, the whole scenario, the whole reality of tomorrow being each time slightly different.

And, knowing full well the future that *will* be will *be,* one begins to understand the reason it eludes him.

The future that *will* be has simply not yet been determined.

It has not yet been decided—however the rigorous chain of cause and effect argues to the contrary that all is *pre*determined. For what predetermination governs the system in which we exist could only be perceptible to someone outside our own dimensional bounds. To a theoretical observer whose perception, being external, was independent of the positional illusions that time and space impose.

Within the system, the only meaningful reality is that which we ourselves perceive.

And one of those realities is the access to choice in a variety of matters—through the exercise of which we, in effect, select the consequences of our acts. Thus, constantly, do we design, create, and furnish with accoutrements the sanctum of the future.

Whether we like it or not—and however the outside observer might disagree—the future-to-be cannot be foreseen simply because we have not fully made up our minds what kind of a place we want it to be.

Nor can we skirt the issue. Back our way into the future, as it were. By default, as a lower animal would, simply *let* it happen. We could not do that if we tried. There are too many predictably achievable accoutrements that we desire.

Even utopia—given its attainment—would, sustained, become old hat. Grown stagnant, would no longer be utopia. Would signal its own destruction.

There is not even a future—automatic in the absence of desire—that will and must happen if no one knows that it is going to. Man *does* know. Within certain limits, that is to say, he has a highly intelligent inkling of the probabilities in store. And try he must, else deny his very nature, to exploit or circumvent them.

In that half-lit sanctum beyond the keyhole, then, what *was* it that we saw? For every feature, scene after reeling scene, was almost palpably authentic. Each scenario as seemingly warm and intimate as any detail in the more familiar substance all around us of the here and now.

What we were seeing, of course, were the options. The myriad futures any one of which we *could* have—*if*.

One for the choosing. And, whether in deliberation or in ignorance, the choice *will* be made.

It will be made by those who, opting not to "meddle" with the future, affect it anyway—inescapably, however innocent of purpose—in everything they do. Just as it will be made—though no more decisively for acts of commission carry no more weight than do acts of overt omission—by those who, with or without reasons of self-interest, spend a fair amount of time in keyhole gazing.

How much to our liking a future is once we are in it, however, is something else again. For we are far more likely to get what we want if we know beforehand the gamut of feasible choices. And that, of course, is what that science-art called "forecasting" is all about. Its purpose, purely and simply, is to bring into view every single option—every single scenario—that we may have the benefit, however we decide, of the widest possible comparison of choices.

At least with respect to the affairs of men, a prediction, then, is merely a statement of *if*. It says in effect, "By such and such a time such and such a thing *could* happen."

Not *will* happen. *Could.*

Whether or not it will happen by the estimated date—for predictions are concerned primarily with *when, any*thing theoretically being possible *in time*—depends in large measure, of course, on whether or not, at the given moment, society opts to go in that particular direction.

Not that the choice is so simply made. Different people at different times want different things. And there is a finite limit to the money, expertise and raw materials that the human ecosystem can ante up at any one time.

In the marketplace of promised wares everything competes. The cure for leukemia must vie with the acquisition of land for parks, with better schooling, with things purported necessary to the national defense —even with such panaceas as heart transplantations and artificial kidneys. All of them in competition for the same potential vendors—tomorrow's crop of experts—the same budget, and the same caches of a biosphere grown noticeably tired of late.

Moreover, concensus takes time, and compromise is never 100 percent to anyone's satisfaction. Yet ultimately societal decisions must and do evolve. With or without—but increasingly *with*—the benefit of keyhole guidance. For as our system's increasing complexity draws on its slack, there is ever less margin for error. Hence, there is an ever greater need to recognize all of the options, and to choose with care.

In the treatment and prevention of human maladies alone, so many options have been forecast that their individual description would be a major dissertation in itself. Taken together, however, they leave one with an unavoidable impression. Within the next three decades—possibly in two decades, conceivably in one —the common inherited maladies of man could be subjected to the onslaught of such weaponry as the last 10,000 decades, the entire span of modern man's existence, could not produce.

And such of those as we opt for, through that massive process of evolving societal druthers, seem likely to fall into every one of the three conventional categories of attack: *euthenics, euphenics* and *eugenics,* plus an esoteric fourth which is totally new—a right-to-the-heart-of-the-problem approach: *gene therapy.*

Though they differ in target and technique, all four approaches have the same objective: to prevent an adverse gene from creating any havoc.

Consider the various ways in which that could conceivably be done.

One could, for example, deprive a gene of the environmental elements it needs to express itself adversely. It is a well known trick, the euthenic approach, incorporating such familiar tactics as the chlorination of water supplies in deference to man's genetic susceptibility to typhoid and the like; minimizing stress in the environs of those who are prone to mental illness; and reducing, through the use of certain environmental props, the spread of streptococci to prevent rheumatic fever.

The elimination from the individual environment of all those provocations that result in malformed infants, say—or of hemolytic crises in those who are G6PD deficient—or of sickle-cell crises in children with sickle-cell anemia—all those will be euthenic too. When they come. Which they could indeed. For they are all there now, in one scenario or another—options.

By the euphenic approach, one avoids the handicaps heredity imposes by making certain compensations to an individual for a gene's adverse expression. Euphenic measures thus include such things as glasses for myopia; insulin medication for the diabetic who cannot make his own; vaccinations against infection; penicillin for bacterial invasion, which invasion is in itself evidence of individual proneness; organ transplantation; psychotherapy; treatment of *any* kind.

Those myriad scenarios, of course, abound with euphenic options, with new or better treatment for a wide variety of ills.

Where will the choice be made?

And on what basis?

Economic perhaps?—with top priority going to those disorders causing the highest man-hour losses in productivity each year along with those that cost the most to care for?

Humanitarian, perhaps?—with priority going primarily to those disorders whose victims, being youngest, have the most to lose?

Or on the basis possibly of fear, with those disorders being emphasized that people as a whole, including those whom we elect to make such final policy decisions, are most afraid of getting?

Or even for reasons academic, the rare, exotic maladies thereby being spared the obvious disadvantage their scarcity would ordinarily impose?

One thing is certain. The problem is not a poverty

of options, it is how to select from among them. And consciously or otherwise, by silence or overt expression, with or without clear conscience, the selection will be made. By each of us, in his own way.

Still another means of circumventing an adverse gene is to deprive it of a host. This is the *eugenic* approach, and the oldest one of all, for it is the method nature uses herself.

Eugenicist she is on every occasion she denies the carrier of an adverse gene the chance to reach—or, if reaching, to take advantage of—reproductive age.

So does man employ eugenics each time, in deference to some flaw in his heredity, he voluntarily abstains from having children. History, recent history at least, is full of such conscientious abstainers. Individuals who in their self-denial, it could be argued, are the real parents of tomorrow. Having helped to shape the future aggregate of human genes as surely as anyone else, they also add to the total human heritage an extra element of conscience. For those who abstain, in general, do so for the *child's* sake, while those who indulge can rarely if ever make any such claim.

The problem with nonprocreation of course—and with artificial insemination, too, as another eugenic technique—is that many an individual who would seriously consider either method has no way of knowing before procreation whether or not the genes he carries could have serious repercussions in his children. And in this regard, the future is as generous as it is with treatment options. For the detection of carriers of a wide variey of deleterious genes—including almost every gene known to result in a metabolic error—now seems achievable by the time this year's crop of children is old enough to vote.

And while no estimated date has been forecast yet for a means of culling from a parent's ova or sperm those that spell genetic trouble, techniques for diagnosing and terminating a blighted pregnancy are here already. Techniques that are applicable not only to all major chromosomal errors but to a growing assortment of metabolic diseases as well.

The number of disorders diagnosable before birth could be doubled—is increasing already, could be tripled—could eventually, perhaps, include even such common lethal maladies, it is said, as sickle-cell anemia. *Could*—again, as always—depending on where society puts its druthers.

And then, of course, there is that right-to-the-crux-of-the-matter approach, gene therapy. In this approach, he who is disadvantaged by a gene that does not work the way it should would be supplied with a gene that does.

Now equipping a cell with an extra gene is actually no trick. It is just that man himself has not yet mastered the technique. Viruses do it routinely, as a way—as a necessity, in fact—of life.

And how *simple* a creature a virus is. No more than a string of genes, naked viral genes, protected from the hostile elements of its would-be host by a raccoon-like protein coat. No more than a miniscule blueprint traveling incognito. Gaining access to the cells of its host, casting off its coat, it strips the cells' own genes of their power and puts all cellular factories to work doing its own genetic bidding. An act of cellular subversion, pure and simple. A genetic *coup d'etat.*

The sniffles of a common cold, then, are in reality but the modest outward signs of a masterful feat of genetic engineering.

Let he whose territorial instinct bristles at the thought, however, ponder it a minute, in an opportunistic frame.

Suppose—just suppose—a virus, say a harmless sort, were to carry a particular gene which the host it "infects," through a stroke of bad hereditary luck, happened to be without. And that just by chance that gene should happen—in the swapping of loyalties that sometimes occurs between the genes of a cell and the genes of its invader—to defect to the other side, becoming a corporate member, a permanent part, of the *cell's* genetic team.

Far-fetched?

Consider the current situation. For as of now every indication says that such a thing is possible. Put certain cells and certain viruses together in a test tube and what happens? A given virus, on entering a cell and taking over, commandeers the manufacture of myriad viral progeny in its own image—which subsequently leave the cell in droves, of course, to stake out cellular territories of their own.

That is the rule.

But exceptions occur.

Every so often—as a result of that cellular chaos that can leave a normally loyal gene confused as to whom it belongs—a viral progeny is born with some of its viral parent's genes and some of the genes of its wet nurse host. A hybrid virus—synthetic, so to speak —often far more like the nurturing cell than like its

viral parent. In essence but a string of escapee cellular
genes—on the loose—free to travel where it will inside
a furry viral coat. Free, by virtue of that coat, to "in-
fect," as it were, whatever species of creature the original virus could.

To a creature host whose cells were deficient in
any gene the invader introduced, such an "infection"
could, of course, be highly consequential. For some of
its cells might just be fortunate enough, via chance de-
fections, to capture the gene in question.

And so it does happen. At least when man deliberately sets the stage.

There are cases on record. Creatures with hereditary defects have, on exposure to certain viral hybrids,
actually been permanently cured. Wee creatures. Only
the very smallest as yet. Bacteria. Those one-celled
beings who, like man, are subject both to adverse genes
and viral parasites.

Could the technique then possibly be made to work
in man himself?

No one is sure. Though the obstacles so far foreseen, it is felt, are all of a solvable sort.

Nor can one be sure, if the method worked, that a
permanent cure would necessarily result. That, of
course, would require that the entering gene be inte-
grated physically into a cell's genetic team, that the cell
be of a long-lived type, and that the integration occur
in *enough* of such cells to meet the body's needs. Otherwise, the gene could be of service to its new-found host
perhaps no longer than the term of the infection, and
periodic readministration would be required to sustain
its effect.

The diabetic mice on whom the technique is already slated for trial—along with mice and rats with certain other metabolic errors that man is also prey to —should soon provide us with some answers.

Meanwhile other techniques have also been suggested. Like coercing cells to forfeit a certain desired gene, for example—all within the province of a test tube—to the cells of an individual in whom that gene is lacking. An actual instance has already been reported. In a recent laboratory trial, the cell of a chicken bequeathed to its test tube mate—the cell from a genetically deficient mouse—the gene the latter lacked.

If such a "take" could be achieved with gene-deficient *human* cells—so the hypothesis goes—their reintroduction into the ailing donor might, like the hybrid virus, conceivably result in a genetic cure.

Still another approach, of course, is the direct transplantation to a gene-deficient human of a small amount of tissue from a nondeficient human. In such a case, one would somehow have to circumvent the body's natural tendency to reject any tissue not intrinsically its own. But even that problem, as progress to date in the entire field of organ transplantation indicates, is apparently not beyond acceptable solution.

True, gene therapy, as currently envisioned, would not prevent an adverse gene from being transmitted to one's children. But the potential application of such therapy appears to be enormous. For any and all disorders due to the lack of one or more normally functioning genes should, theoretically at least, be amenable to such treatment.

Moreover the predictions grow shorter, not longer. Treatment or cure of certain metabolic defects with the proper doses of the proper genes may now be possible, it is suggested, not in fifty or one hundred years but in ten, or even five. If valid, such an assessment would seem to indicate that society has opted already to pursue a course in which gene therapy might well become the major feature in the treatment of the bulk of our really disabling gene-based ills.

Ironically, it is the likely success of all such measures, from gene therapy to euthenics, combined of course with the myriad treatment procedures already in existence, that creates—according to a growing number of concerned observers—an unparalleled human dilemma.

Each new technique that enables a greater number of those with a given defect to reach or take advantage of the reproductive years increases the frequency of the gene at fault in the population's gene pool.

Normally, within that pool, there is a balance of sorts in that the carriers of an adverse gene, by failing to reproduce, take the gene out of circulation about as fast as fresh mutations, in other families, put it back.

Now ever since man first took upon himself the job of caring for his sick—likely fifty thousand years ago at least—he has been interfering with that balance. Even the simple act of feeding those too weak with one acute infection or another to feed themselves must surely have increased the survival of the more infection-prone among him. And how serious an infection is —typhoid, smallpox, or what have you—does vary from one individual to another in part on genetic grounds.

Nothing in man's past history, of course, can

match the therapeutic explosion of the last fifty years. Nor has the frequency, of late, of many an adverse gene, in the aftermath of a new technique, been allowed to plateau at a higher level in the gene pool of our species before another new technique sends it climbing again.

And it is that pool, after all, that each coming generation, in its turn, must draw on, blindly, for its own supply of genes.

There is, for example, little doubt that the frequency of diabetic genes took a sudden jump in the first forty years after insulin's introduction. Or that epilepsy genes have increased somewhat since the advent of effective anti-convulsant treatment. Likewise, rheumatic fever genes in the wake of penicillin—even certain "birth defect genes" which once, before modern surgery, and if only on cosmetic grounds, played havoc with one's reproductive chances.

So might one expect that, at this very moment, the frequency of genes for schizophrenia, for manic-depressive psychosis, for sickle-cell anemia—for any disease which strikes before or during reproductive age and for which effective treatment has only lately begun to take shape—is quietly starting to climb. A quiet, however, which will almost surely be broken by time and the inexorable momentum of successive generations.

However resolvable, in whatever way, the dilemma is real.

To indulge the present, it would seem, denies the future. To indulge the future perforce denies the present.

Where is the solution?

That is the question which those who are truly concerned would raise as the primary issue.

Their concern, of course, is based largely on assumptions.

The first such assumption is that future changes in the environment will not recast such genes in a role more beneficial—an assumption which probability, admittedly, does seem to favor.

The second is that the resources for treating such afflictions may not keep pace with increasing demands —a possibility to some extent supported by the lack of tangible assurance to the contrary.

The third is that a failure to stem the increase of adverse genes might sooner or later force us, whether or not we wanted, to opt for the test tube in place of the family as a procreating unit. The likelihood of that, however, is hard to assess in view of the capacity of human beings, now and then at least, to hold certain fates to be worse than even that ultimate state of not being here to have options at all.

The last is that there is some unassailable reason why the human species *must not* go to pot. This assumption—however unfounded, for the point is moot —does at least have the virtue of providing man with an extra sense of purpose.

The expressed concern, then, is not without some foundation. And those who confess to such qualms are also quick to point to certain realities of life that argue, they say, against the problem's disappearing on its own.

One reality is man's commitment—as basic to his nature as any of his genes—to care for his kind. Those who are here and hurting now cannot be denied. Within the limits of our wherewithal to meet that need, however predetermined that may be by other competing human needs, there is no question that he who stands to benefit from treatment must and shall receive it. No service to the yet unborn accrues from dehumanizing tactics, for tactics themselves are passed along as readily as genes.

Another reality is the normal human resistance to radical change. The last resort in human quality control—societally regulated test tube births—is so vastly different from the life styles anyone is familiar with that the majority of people would likely prefer even species deterioration.

Still another reality is the understandable difficulty people have in denying themselves, for the social good, the satisfaction of having children when the total effect of any one of them, as an individual parent, is so small. It is the same kind of rationale as that which keeps many a would-be voter from the polls on election day —or allows the occasional individual truly concerned about overpopulation to wind up—somehow—with half a dozen children. Or those who worry about air pollution to desist wherever possible from using public transportation.

Inherent in that expressed concern with the gene pool, of course, is the seed of a delicate issue.

The right to bear a child.

To be sure, it is not so delicate an issue that man has never had the courage to express himself on the matter.

Laws forbidding the epileptic to marry state, however implicitly, that certain individuals do *not* have the right to children.

The last of such laws, it is true, disappeared from the books three years ago. But their repeal was due not so much to a public sense of having trampled on sacred ground as to a growing realization of the decision's arbitrary nature, having been made entirely out of context with no consideration being given other inherited disorders, having been motivated by concern with superficial appearance rather than with disability *per se,* and, finally, having been arrived at with few genetic salients at hand.

The right-to-children issue, of course, resolves to the more specific question—when does the individual right to children become subordinate to mankind's right to a certain level of quality defined in terms of health?

Never? Even if the species should deteriorate as a result to a point where the laws of the jungle—the mandates of brutish natural selection—begin on their own to try to rectify matters?

Or, if a contest can indeed be granted between the individual and his species in which the latter, like the former, is entitled to some protection by certain basic rules, what *kind* of rules? And when will they be applied? Now or not until the problem becomes truly manifest as such? And to *whom* will they apply? In what situations? And at what level of compromise between the two contestants?

Three things only seem relatively certain.

The answers *will* emerge. Even ignoring the matter cannot ward the answers off, for turning one's back

to the issue simply acts as a vote in favor of those who
opt instead to face it.

The second certainty, and apropos of the first, is
that such answers will not be established by any special
interest group, including scientists *per se*. Nor by elitist
panels. Nor—as those who would shun participation
sometimes fearfully complain—by "totalitarians" in
our midst.

They will be the product exclusively of that herculean smith who forges social policy across the board
—*public opinion*. The amalgamation, as it were, of
individual druthers, fashioned from the gossamer substance of human values and perceptions. For the answer to any question concerning human rights has
never a basis in fact. It is a matter of individual—of
personal—opinion. No more, no less.

Even those who claim to be backed by one or another form of Absolute, when the count is taken, can
speak only for themselves. As must also those whose
sense of rightness derives instead from the irrefutabili-
ties of secular statistics. For no man yet has been voluntarily given by his fellow men the privilege of putting
words into someone else's unconsenting mouth.

The final certainty has to do with the temporal
nature of everything man does. However the issue is
resolved today—by whatever values and perceptions
—no lasting attitude is necessarily assured. Nothing is
forever. Every generation reserves the right to judge
anew—to patch, repair, expand, undo and recreate.

Human rights, with time, are constantly redefined
—as changes in our hardware and our software beget
and are begot by changes in our values.

It is necessarily so. However we might like to envision the future in the image of the present—to assure ad infinitum its conformance to the standards and the mores we hold dear—we should like it not at all had we ourselves been so restricted by prehistoric forebears who foresaw the disregard with which we were to dispossess ourselves of their most cherished notions and possessions.

One final word—lest one worry that man is too naive, too inexperienced in matters of evolutionary peril, either to comprehend completely or, with any degree of expertise, to cope with problems of the ilk the gene pool seems to be posing.

He is nothing of the sort. For dilemma always was, and always will be, par for the human course.

Human history is entirely a log of critical decisions. And if problems grow increasingly complex with time, it can only be that we, as creatures of our culture, have ourselves become sufficiently complex to make them so. And hence, theoretically at least, sufficiently complex to render their solution.

It is doubtful, moreover—however perilous the human course might seem to be—that man would have it any other way.

There is nothing, at any rate, in his prevailing attitudes and actions to suggest that he would alter his direction if he could—strange as that may seem, for he is, in a sense, in a predicament from which there is little hope of extrication.

Picture his plight. It takes but little imagination to conjure up the scene.

Contemporary man, midsea in evolutionary sojourn—out on some reefy stepping stone, as it were, the latest in the course of his genetic-cultural progression—pausing now, as always, to take another sighting.

Behind, in the dark millennial waters between himself and the animal shore of his departure, the reefy perches that one by one provided him with footing in the past—with the very foundation of his previous existence—have long ago disappeared.

Only now and then between the swells ahead can he glimpse the misty outline of the opposite shore. That one whose only reality he alone must give it—if indeed, receding ahead of him as it usually seems to be, it will ever be there at all.

Beneath his feet the reef that gives him his contemporary footing is already starting to shift. Unavoidably, under his restless weight, to tilt like the others and sink.

Within his leaping reach the reef ahead looms like an invitation, half-phantom in the mist. And well he knows he cannot tarry where he is.

One false step, one miscalculation, and only the roily water will mark his journey's end.

A suspenseful scene. One that would surely make nature herself—had she the eyes to see her venturesome child in his perennial state of peril—hold her breath and in a throe of maternal guilt reproach herself for ever having let him stray offshore.

Too late.

All her maternal prevailings could not deter him now. Beladen with the problems his own rash freedom has begot, undaunted by their weight, by the risks their very solution must involve, he is obsessed. From any other viewpoint than his own, a traveler taken leave of his senses.

For like those legendary mariners of old who, on hearing the sirens' song, were compelled in their direction without regard to peril, he is bewitched by the sound of singing in the mists ahead.

Music he is powerless to resist.

Such haunting strains as only sheer nostalgia for what has yet to be could have inspired. Song ringing with the promise, as it were, of all the things that must forever lie beyond what lies beyond. Of destiny perpetually in motion.

But the voice he hears—compelling as the sirens'—is naught but the lingering sound of his echo in the mist.

And the song, that too, is his own.

Index

Achondroplastic dwarfism, 6, 11

Allergy, 191

Anemia, 73–93; *see also* Sickle cell anemia and G6PD deficiency

Anisometropia, *see* Mixed errors of refraction

Ankylosing spondylitis, 39–44; detection, 43; genetics, 40; occurrence, 40; prevalence, 40; prevention, 42–43; risk of inheritance, 41–42

Amblyopia: in mixed errors of refraction, 67; in squint, 68, 69

Arthritis, 31–52; prevalence, 32; *see also* Ankylosing spondylitis, Gout, Osteoarthritis, and Rheumatoid arthritis

Astigmatism, 65; genetics, 65; prevalence, 65; risk of inheritance, 65

Birth defects, 151–163; cleft palate, 154; club foot, 154; environmental factors in, 152; genetic factors in, 152–153; harelip, 153–154; heart defects, 155; multiple defects, 155; prevalence, 151; prevention, 155; pyloric stenosis, 154–155; spina bifida, 154; *see also* Hip dislocation, Urinary system malformations

Cancer, 181–185; breast, 181–182; environmental factors in, 183–184; genetic factors in, 181–183; leukemia, 182; lung, 182; other common cancers, 182–183; stomach, 182

Cataract, 57–63; genetic factors in, 57–58, 59; prevention, 58, 61; risk of inheritance, 59, 60
Cerebral palsy, 180
Coronary heart disease, 185–188; diabetes and, 187; environmental factors in, 186; genetic factors in, 186–188; high blood pressure and, 187; metabolic defects and, 187; prevalence, 185; prevention, 188
Crossed eyes, *see* Squint

Diabetes, 15–29; detection, 25–26; environmental factors in, 26–27; genetic factors in, 15–16; history, 18–22; in coronary heart disease, 187; prevalence, 17–18; prevention, 25–27; risk of inheritance, 23–25
Dislocation of hip, *see* Hip Dislocation
Disorders of hearing, *see* Otosclerosis
Disorders of vision, *see* Visual disorders
Down's disease, *see* Mongolism

Emphysema, 188–189; environmental factors in, 189; genetic factors in, 189; prevalence, 189; prevention, 190
Epilepsy, 121–137; detection, 130; environmental factors in, 126–127, 130; genetic factors in, 128–130, 133; prevalence,

126; prevention, 134–135; relationship to migraine, 136; risk of inheritance, 130–132, 134
Eugenics, 198, 200, 201
Euphenics, 198, 199
Euthenics, 198

Farsightedness, 64–65; genetic factors in, 64; prevention, 64; risk of inheritance, 64

G6PD deficiency, 85–93; basic defect in, 87–88; detection, 92; environmental factors in, 85, 88–89; genetic factors in, 89–92; history, 85–87; occurrence, 87; prevalence, 87; prevention, 88, 91, 92; relationship to malaria, 86; risk of inheritance, 90–92
Gene therapy, 198, 201–204
Glaucoma, 68–72; detection, 71; genetic factors in, 70; prevention, 71; risk of inheritance, 70–71
Goitre, 180
Gout, 44–52; detection, 48–50; genetic factors in, 47; history, 44–46; occurrence, 47, 51; prevention, 48–50; risk of inheritance, 47–48

Hearing loss, *see* Otosclerosis
Heart disease, *see* Rheumatic fever, Coronary heart disease
Heberden's nodes, 36–37;

environmental factors in, 36; genetic factors in, 37; occurrence, 37; prevention, 37–38; risk of inheritance, 37

High blood pressure, *see* Hypertension

Hip dislocation, 156–159; basic defect, 156; detection, 157; environmental factors in, 157, 158, 159; genetic factors in, 156; occurrence, 156; prevention, 157–158; risk of inheritance, 157

Hypertension, 187

Huntington's chorea, 7, 11–12

Hyperopia, *see* Farsightedness

Malformations, *see* Birth defects

Malformations of the urinary system, *see* Urinary system malformations

Manic-depressive psychosis, 100–103; detection, 102; genetic factors in, 101; prevalence, 101; prevention, 102–103; risk of inheritance, 101–102

Mental illness, 95–100; mimicry by drugs, 95–96; *see also* Manic-depressive psychosis, Schizophrenia

Mental retardation, 156–178; environmental factors in, 167–168; genetic factors in, 168; prevalence, 167; risk of inheritance, 161; *see also* Mongolism

Mixed errors of refraction, 66–67; genetic factors in, 67; prevention, 67

Mongolism, 168–178; basic defect, 169–171, 174–175; detection, 176–177; effects of maternal age, 171, 174; environmental factors in, 171–172; prevalence, 168; prevention, 177; risk of inheritance, 172–175

Muscular dystrophy, 5

Myopia, *see* Nearsightedness

Nearsightedness, 65–66; genetic factors in, 65; prevention, 65; risks of inheritance, 65

Neurofibromatosis, 7–8

Osteoarthritis, 35–39; environmental factors in, 36, 38; genetic factors in, 36; occurrence, 35–36; prevalence, 39; prevention, 38–39

Otosclerosis, 191

Rh disease of infants: environmental factors in, 145–146; genetic factors in, 144; prevalence, 145; prevention, 147–149; risk of inheritance, 147

Rheumatic fever, 111–120; detection, 115; environmental factors in, 112, 118–120; genetic factors in, 114; occurrence, 111, 113, 115;

Rheumatic Fever (continued)
prevalence, 111, 112; prevention, 115–118; risk of
inheritance, 114–115

Schizophrenia, 104–110;
detection, 108; environmental
factors in, 108; genetic factors
in, 104–107; occurrence, 104,
105; prevalence, 104; prevention, 108–109; risk of inheritance, 107–108
Sickle cell anemia, 75–85; basic
defect, 75–78; detection, 81;
environmental factors in, 79;
genetic factors in, 78; history,
82–84; occurrence, 78–79;
prevalence of cases, 78–79;
    prevalence of carriers, 79;

prevention, 81–82; relationship to malaria, 82–83; risk
of inheritance, 80–81;
symptoms in the carrier state,
82
Squint, 68–70; genetic factors
in, 63; farsightedness and,
64–65; nearsightedness and,
66; prevalence, 62; prevention,
63; risk of inheritance, 63

Urinary system malformations,
159–162; detection, 161;
genetic factors in, 160;
prevalence, 159; prevention,
161; risk of inheritance, 160

Visual disorders, 53–72; *see also
disorders by name*